Practice Examination Papers for the MRCPsych Part 1

Sabina Burza
North London SHO Training Scheme in Psychiatry

with

Beata Mougey
North London SHO Training Scheme in Psychiatry

Srinivas Perecherla
St Mary's, London SHO Training Scheme in Psychiatry

and

Nakul Talwar
St Mary's, London SHO Training Scheme in Psychiatry

T0138951

Radcliffe Publishing
Oxford ● Seattle

Radcliffe Publishing Ltd
18 Marcham Road
Abingdon
Oxon OX14 1AA
United Kingdom

www.radcliffe-oxford.com
Electronic catalogue and worldwide online ordering facility.

British Library Cataloguing in Publication Data

A catalogue record for this book is available from the British Library.

ISBN 1 85775 668 1

Typeset by Advance Typesetting Ltd, Oxford
Printed and bound by TJ International Ltd, Padstow, Cornwall

Contents

Foreword

Multiple-choice questions, which for many years were the principal method for assessing knowledge in the MRCPsych written examination, were never popular. The rigid format of one stem and five 'true' or 'false' responses made them frustrating to write and even more frustrating to try to answer. The requirement to find five items on the same topic often meant that obscure material had to be dredged in order to complete a whole question. For instance, psychiatrists should know that Huntington's chorea is an autosomal dominant condition. After a few months of revision many will know that neurofibromatosis and polycystic kidney disease are as well. But do we really need to know the names of the hundreds of other rare conditions that have sometimes worked their way into MCQs?

The Royal College of Psychiatrists has now dropped MCQs from the MRCPsych examination – I suspect there will be few who will be sad to see them go. In their place have come new formats such as individual statements (IS) and extended matching items (EMIs). No method for testing a person's knowledge is perfect, not least because the information that underpins this knowledge is less precise and stable than is often recognised. However, individual statements should enable salient issues to be considered without the baggage of other less relevant items, and EMIs provide an opportunity to test reasoning as well as the accumulation of facts.

Exam practice books have always provided an important means of helping candidates to prepare for written papers. After several weeks of reading textbooks and papers they can also provide a way of making revision more interesting and varied. This book by four psychiatrists in training is based on their first-hand experience of preparing for (and passing!) their membership exams. The book provides one of the first collections of psychiatry questions that focus on individual statements and extended matching items. In producing a comprehensive collection of these types of question and covering the full range of topics encountered in the MRCPsych, the authors have produced a book that will be of great value to all those preparing for postgraduate examinations in psychiatry. I am pleased to have the opportunity to recommend it as a revision aid for psychiatrists in training.

Dr Mike Crawford
Senior Lecturer in Psychiatry
Department of Psychological Medicine
Faculty of Medicine, Imperial College London
April 2005

Preface

The MRCPsych Part 1 has recently undergone changes in format. All four authors, having sat the Part 1 examination in spring 2003, were among the first group of candidates to be exposed to the recent alterations. The lack of updated revision aids at that time was infuriating, and germinated the idea for this book.

Although this situation has since changed, there continues to be a lack of books that reflect the actual exam format, despite the fact that practice papers under timed conditions form a vital part of successful preparation. Therefore this book can be used not only by those early on in their revision, as a source of learning (we know that often this is a much preferred method to opening a huge tome!), but also by those later on in their revision who wish to sit simulated exams.

Each of the four chapters consists of a practice paper together with answers and explanations. These reflect the new format of 133 individual statements (IS) together with extended matching items (EMIs) worth 67 marks in total for each paper. The breakdown of questions from the different subjects reflects that of the actual exam; further information on this can be obtained from the college website at www.rcpsych.ac.uk. We have included references for each answer, as we are well aware of the sometimes infuriating differences in opinion between sources. These references can also function as a source of further reading.

We are grateful to all those who helped with the preparation of the book, and we would like to thank Sakib Burza and, in particular, Borzoueh Mohammadi for their unending support and assistance.

Sabina Burza
April 2005

About the authors

Sabina Burza MRCPsych graduated from Cambridge University and the Royal Free Hospital School of Medicine in the late 1990s and subsequently trained on the North London SHO scheme in psychiatry. **Nakul Talwar** MRCPsych is a graduate of University College Hospital and has since been a trainee on the St Mary's SHO rotation. **Sri Perecherla** MRCPsych and **Beata Mougey** are overseas graduates from Osmania Medical College, Hyderabad, India and Silician Medical Academy in Katowice, Poland, respectively. Sri is also a trainee on the St Mary's rotation, and Beata is on the North London rotation. Currently all four authors work in psychiatric sub-specialities within London.

List of abbreviations

BBB	blood–brain barrier
BMI	body mass index
BP	blood pressure
CJD	Creutzfeld–Jacob disease
CK	creatinine kinase
CNS	central nervous system
COMT	catechol-O-methyltransferase
CR	conditioned response
CS	conditioned stimulus
CSF	cerebrospinal fluid
CT	computerised tomography
CVA	cerebrovascular accident
DA	dopamine
DOPAC	dihydroxyphenylacetic acid
DSH	deliberate self-harm
DSM-IV	*Diagnostic and Statistical Manual of Mental Disorders*, fourth edition
ECG	electrocardiogram
ECT	electroconvulsive therapy
EEG	electroencephalogram
EPSE	extrapyramidal side-effects
FBC	full blood count
FRS	first-rank symptoms
GABA	gamma-aminobutyric acid
GFR	glomerular filtration rate
GHQ	General Health Questionnaire
GI	gastrointestinal
HVA	homovanillic acid
IUGR	intrauterine growth retardation
LFT	liver function test

LMN	lower motor neuron
LSD	lysergic acid diethylamide
LTM	long-term memory
MAO	monoamine oxidase
MAOI	monoamine oxidase inhibitor
MDMA	3,4-methylenedioxymethamphetamine
MHPG	3-methoxy-4-hydroxyphenylglycol
MS	multiple sclerosis
NARI	noradrenaline reuptake inhibitor
NMDA	N-methyl-D-aspartate
OCD	obsessive-compulsive disorder
OPC	outpatient clinic
PANSS	Positive and Negative Symptoms Scale
PD	personality disorder
PSE	Present State Examination
PTSD	post-traumatic stress disorder
RCT	randomised controlled trial
REM	rapid eye movement
SCID	structured clinical interview for DSM-IV
SSRI	selective serotonin reuptake inhibitor
TCA	tricyclic antidepressant
TD	tardive dyskinesia
TRH	thyroid-releasing hormone
TSH	thyroid-stimulating hormone
UCR	unconditioned response
UCS	unconditioned stimulus
UMN	upper motor neuron
VMA	vanillyl mandelic acid
WAIS	Weschler Adult Intelligence Scale
WHO	World Health Organization
YBOCS	Yale–Brown Obsessive-Compulsive Scale
5-HIAA	5-hydroxyindoleacetic acid
5HT	5-hydroxytryptamine

Paper 1:
Questions

Q1 Perceptual set refers to the readiness to perceive particular features of a stimulus.

Q2 Nomothetic theories of personality are concerned with trait and type theories.

Q3 The halo effect means that personal space needs to be maintained when one is around others.

Q4 Interpersonal attraction is enhanced by dissimilarity.

Q5 Social exchange theory views people as fundamentally selfish and concerned with the least expense–gain ratio in any relationship.

Q6 A bystander in an emergency blames the victim to reduce cognitive dissonance.

Q7 Two of the specific effects of TV violence are arousal and inhibition.

Q8 Conformity decreases with increasing group number.

Q9 According to Milgram, a participant's obedience is increased in the presence of an experimenter.

Q10 The Stanford–Binet test includes subtests of short-term memory and reasoning.

Q11 Block design is a performance subtest of the WAIS.

Q12 Fluid intelligence relates to specific knowledge acquired through life.

Q13 Believing that 'bad things happen to people because they themselves are bad' is an example of the fundamental attribution error.

Q14 According to Freud, the theory of moral development consists of six developmental stages categorised into three levels.

Q15 According to Piaget, accommodation refers to the incorporation of new information into schemas.

Q16 Nurturing parents with low expectations have an authoritative parenting style.

Q17 Gender constancy is usually achieved by the age of 5 years.

Q18 In terms of emotional support men benefit more from marriage than women.

Q19 With increasing age there is usually no decline in semantic memory but a slight decline in episodic memory.

Q20 Stranger anxiety in children usually appears at 2 years of age.

Q21 Individuals who experienced physical abuse in childhood are less likely to repeat abusive behaviours towards their own children.

Q22 Respondent learning, also known as classical conditioning, is learned suddenly after one trial.

Q23 In second-order conditioning, a conditioned stimulus acts as an unconditioned stimulus.

(Q24) In contrast to depth perception, figure ground differentiation and perceptual constancy are innate.

(Q25) Dual-task interference refers to the impaired attention that occurs when attending to two sources of information simultaneously.

(Q26) Approximately 15% of children have an eidetic memory.

(Q27) The maximum number of items that can be stored in working memory is nine.

(Q28) Proactive interference refers to the phenomenon whereby new learning impairs information that has already been learned.

(Q29) The Yerkes–Dodson curve is an inverted U-shape.

(Q30) Hyperthermia increases blood–brain barrier permeability.

(Q31) ECT decreases the permeability of the blood–brain barrier.

(Q32) Phenytoin is a lipophilic drug.

(Q33) Drugs with zero-order kinetics are more likely to cause toxic reactions than those with first-order kinetics.

(Q34) Alcohol follows both zero- and first-order kinetics.

(Q35) Fluoxetine increases the level of TCAs.

(Q36) The volume of distribution of drugs in the elderly is affected by their decreased body fat.

(Q37) Carbamazepine may cause both constipation and diarrhoea.

(Q38) Chlorpromazine rarely causes extrapyramidal symptoms.

(Q39) Extrapyramidal symptoms are more common with trifluoperazine than with chlorpromazine.

(Q40) Priapism is a known adverse effect of clozapine.

(Q41) Lithium may cause blurred vision at therapeutic doses.

(Q42) Lofepramine is not cardiotoxic in overdose.

(Q43) The ECGs of patients on TCAs frequently show prolongation of the PR and QT intervals.

(Q44) In toxic doses TCAs may cause bradycardia, but not tachycardia.

(Q45) Coughing and yawning are known side-effects of citalopram.

(Q46) Fluvoxamine commonly causes postural hypotension.

(Q47) In contrast to the $GABA_A$ receptor, all dopamine receptors are metabotropic.

(Q48) Vigabatrin, an inhibitor of GABA aminotransferase, results in decreased production of GABA.

(Q49) Glutamate, the principal excitatory neurotransmitter in the CNS, is synthesised from glutamine.

(Q50) Venlafaxine has a high affinity for cholinergic and alpha-epinephric receptors.

(Q51) Clomipramine is the TCA that most strongly inhibits the reuptake of 5HT.

(Q52) Reboxetine is a norepinephrine and 5HT reuptake inhibitor.

(Q53) DOPAC and VMA are breakdown products of dopamine.

(Q54) It is thought that ECT results in increased norepinephrine and dopamine activity.

Q55 Carbamazepine induces its own metabolism.

Q56 The term used to describe the adverse effects developed by subjects receiving placebo treatment in a trial is the nocebo effect.

Q57 A placebo that produces side-effects is termed an active placebo.

Q58 Perseveration is a symptom that characteristically occurs in schizophrenia.

Q59 The circadian cycle of a human has a duration of more than 24 hours.

Q60 First-rank symptoms occur only in schizophrenia.

Q61 According to Crow, type II schizophrenia is characterised by delusions and hallucinations.

Q62 Depersonalisation can occur in children.

Q63 Depersonalisation is a recognised symptom of organic states.

Q64 Dysarthria is a symptom of pseudobulbar palsy.

Q65 Cryptolalia is a type of formal thought disorder and occurs only in schizophrenia.

Q66 Individuals with pure word blindness are unable to write.

Q67 Obsessions may occur as thoughts, images or impulses.

Q68 Obsessional images may be vivid and not always recognised as one's own.

Q69 Manic patients are prone to drink too much alcohol, but do not usually overeat.

(Q70) Obesity may be associated with hypoventilation in the Pickwickian syndrome.

(Q71) The essential feature of paranoid personality disorder is self reference.

(Q72) Married people in general suffer more mental illness.

(Q73) Erikson defined Integrity versus Despair as conflicts encountered in early adulthood.

(Q74) Typically, grief resolves within 18–24 months.

(Q75) Primary delusions only occur in schizophrenia.

(Q76) In Cotard's syndrome, it is believed that a familiar person has been replaced by a double.

(Q77) In folie communiqué, separation of the psychotic and non-psychotic individuals results in symptom remission in the latter.

(Q78) Macropsia can occur in parietal lobe lesions.

(Q79) Splitting of perception may occur in schizophrenia.

(Q80) Completion illusions occur when carefully attending to stimuli.

(Q81) Lilliputian hallucinations typically occur in delirium tremens.

(Q82) The most common psychiatric cause of autoscopic hallucinations is schizophrenia.

(Q83) Tactile hallucinations are almost always delusionally elaborated.

(Q84) Delusional significance is the second stage of delusional perception.

Q85 According to Kretschmer, sensitive ideas of reference may develop into delusions in those with a sensitive premorbid personality.

Q86 Chronically delusional patients, compared with those whose delusions have recently remitted, have been shown to score higher for positive meaning in life.

Q87 Sleep drunkenness occurs while falling asleep.

Q88 Megaphagia is a feature of the Kleine–Levin syndrome.

Q89 The preconscious, which serves to maintain the repression of memories contained within the unconscious, can become overpowered in neurosis.

Q90 Freud believed dreams to be composed of the night residue, unconscious wishes and nocturnal stimuli.

Q91 The Electra complex is a phenomenon of the genital stage.

Q92 In terms of Jungian theory, the Anima and Shadow are archetypes.

Q93 The depressive position starts to develop at the age of 18 months.

Q94 Psychodrama is particularly useful for those who have difficulties expressing themselves verbally.

Q95 'I and thou' and 'no gossiping' are principles of gestalt therapy.

Q96 Encounter groups are associated with Carl Rogers.

Q97 Dissociation can be seen as a form of conversion.

Q98 Schizophrenia should not be diagnosed if dysmorphophobia is the first reported symptom.

Q99 Gender identity is normally established by the age of about 18 months.

Q100 The discrepancy between self-image and biological sex in gender identity disorder is usually clearly established only after puberty.

Q101 In paedophilia there is frequently a history of severe psycho-social deprivation during the perpetrator's childhood.

Q102 Suicide is commonly committed by individuals held in custody.

Q103 Individuals completing suicide have been found to have low CSF 5-HIAA levels.

Q104 Depression during pregnancy is associated with an unwanted pregnancy.

Q105 One-third of women develop depression during the post-partum period.

Q106 Lithium is a first-line treatment in rapid cycling affective disorder.

Q107 A good response to lithium is predicted by bipolar illnesses that have manic episodes followed by depression.

Q108 Screening questionnaires in the UK have identified alcohol misuse in up to 30% of all female admissions to general hospitals.

Q109 The risk of alcohol misuse is higher in certain occupational groups, including actors, entertainers and printers.

Q110 Characteristic features of Wernicke's encephalopathy include irritability, severe memory impairment and confabulation.

(Q111) Kretschmer described three types of body build, including pyknic, athletic and asthenic.

(Q112) The prevalence of personality disorders is generally higher in rural than in urban populations.

(Q113) In ICD-10, changes in personality due to organic disease of the brain are classified in the chapter on disorders of adult personality and behaviour.

(Q114) Cushing's syndrome and Addison's disease are recognised causes of fatigue.

(Q115) Boufee delirante is another term for the acute polymorphic psychotic disorders.

(Q116) Bipolar I disorder is characterised by the occurrence of one or more major depressive episodes accompanied by at least one hypomanic episode.

(Q117) Leaden paralysis, according to DSM-IV, is a feature of atypical depression.

(Q118) The presence of biological symptoms is predictive of a good response to ECT.

(Q119) The course of generalised anxiety disorder tends to be constant.

(Q120) The onset of an acute stress reaction is usually within minutes of exposure to an exceptional stressor.

(Q121) Most dissociative states tend to remit after a few weeks or months.

(Q122) Multiple sclerosis is a common cause of frontal lobe syndrome.

Q123 Schizophreniform, schizo-affective and affective psychoses are well recognised complications of temporal lobe epilepsy.

Q124 Knowledge of how to use language is characteristically preserved in the amnesic syndrome.

Q125 Agraphia and agraphaesthesia are interchangeable terms.

Q126 In terms of speech dominance and handedness, 85% of right-handers are left hemisphere dominant.

Q127 Visual hallucinations in dementia are typically non-threatening.

Q128 Personality is relatively well preserved in subcortical dementia.

Q129 The weight-to-weight potency of methadone approximately matches that of morphine.

Q130 Depression is a recognised risk factor for non-compliance with medical treatment.

Q131 Somatic symptoms are reported more often by individuals in developed than in developing countries.

Q132 Hypopituitarism has been associated with improved sexual functioning.

Q133 There are increased rates of schizotypal personality disorder among the relatives of probands with schizophrenia.

EMI 1

Options:

A Extensor plantar reflex
B Flapping tremor
C Intention tremor
D Neck stiffness
E Nystagmus
F Optic atrophy
G Perseveration
H Petechial rash
I Resting tremor
J Urinary hesitancy

For each of the following conditions, choose the **most appropriate** symptom/sign from the list above. The number of answers required for each condition is indicated in parentheses. Each option may be used once, more than once or not at all.

Q134 A 45-year-old man with Wernicke's encephalopathy. (1)

Q135 Following an attack of mastoiditis, a 16-year-old boy develops pyrexia, headache, vomiting and impaired consciousness. (2)

Q136 A 60-year-old man suffering from hepatic encephalopathy. (1)

Q137 A 70-year-old man with Parkinson's disease. (1)

EMI 2

Options:

A Bradycardia
B Bronchospasm
C Confusion
D Hair loss
E Influenza-like symptoms
F Microcytosis
G Myoclonus
H Osteomalacia
I Rash
J Significant weight gain
K Tachycardia

From the above list, choose the **two most likely** side-effects of the medications below. Each option can be used once, more than once or not at all.

(Q138) A young woman taking lamotrigine as a mood stabiliser.

(Q139) A middle-aged man uses propranolol for his symptoms of anxiety.

(Q140) A 30-year-old woman takes sodium valproate and olanzapine concomitantly.

(Q141) A 40-year-old man is prescribed tranylcypromine concurrently with clomipramine.

EMI 3

Options:

A   Beck Depression Inventory
B   Carroll Rating Scale
C   General Health Questionnaire
D   Halstead–Reitan Battery
E   Hamilton Rating Scale for Depression
F   Montgomery–Asberg Depression Rating Scale
G   YBOCS

From the list above, choose the **most appropriate** scale for the following scenarios. **One** answer is required for each question. Each option can be used once, more than once or not at all.

Q142   Identification of psychiatric cases of neurosis in the community.

Q143   Assessment of the psychological and somatic symptoms of depression.

Q144   Assessment specifically for the psychological symptoms of depression.

Q145   Self-rating scale for depressed patients.

Q146   Assessment of severity of brain damage.

EMI 4

Options:

A   Clomipramine
B   Lofepramine
C   Mianserin
D   Phenelzine
E   Reboxetine
F   Trazodone
G   Venlafaxine

For each of the following scenarios, choose the **most appropriate** drug from the list above. Each question requires **one** answer only. Each option can be used once, more than once or not at all.

Q147   A 35-year-old man was started on this antidepressant. He was seen 6 weeks later in the OPC, where he mentioned he had stopped taking the drug as he had developed a painful and prolonged erection.

Q148   A 29-year-old woman was started on this antidepressant. She was asked to have a blood test for an FBC every 4 weeks for the first 3 months.

Q149   A 55-year-old man was started on this TCA, which has been found to be safer in both overdose and cardiovascular disease compared with other TCAs.

Q150   A 34-year-old man was started on this antidepressant, which selectively enhances noradrenaline neurotransmission.

Q151   A 29-year-old woman was started on this antidepressant, which is also indicated for phobic and obsessional states.

EMI 5

Options:

A   Attachment theory
B   Easy child, difficult child, slow to warm up child
C   Ego Integrity versus Despair
D   Theory of moral development
E   Three styles of child rearing
F   Timely death
G   Transitional object
H   Pre-operational stage

For each of the following, choose the **most appropriate** option from the list above. Each question requires **one** answer only. Each option can be used once, more than once or not at all.

Q152   Bowlby.

Q153   Erikson.

Q154   Winnicott.

Q155   Kohlberg.

Q156   Baumrind.

Q157   Thomas and Chess.

Q158   Piaget.

EMI 6

Options:

A Age less than 1 year
B Chomsky's view on language development
C Concrete operational stage
D Eighteen months to 3 years
E Formal operational stage
F Piaget's view on language development
G Pre-operational stage
H Sensorimotor stage
I Skinner's view on language development
J Three years onwards
K Vygotsky's view on language development

For each of the following descriptions, choose the **most appropriate** option from the list above. Each question requires **one** answer only. Each option can be used once, more than once or not at all.

Q159 Possessing a vocabulary of about 300 words.

Q160 Language is believed to be acquired by operant conditioning and parental imitation. Grammar development is thought to be acquired via differential reinforcement.

Q161 Object permanence is acquired during this stage.

Q162 Animism and centration are found in this stage of development.

Q163 Egocentrism and an inability to understand conservation are found in this stage of development.

Q164 Language development is postulated to occur by children building their own schemata via active exploration of their environment.

EMI 7

Options:

A   Chaining
B   Fixed interval schedule
C   Fixed ratio schedule
D   Generalisation
E   Instrumental learning
F   Negative reinforcement
G   Positive reinforcement
H   Punishment
I   Respondent learning
J   Second-order conditioning
K   Shaping
L   Variable interval schedule
M   Variable ratio schedule
N   Vicarious learning

For each of the following scenarios, choose the **most appropriate** option from the list above. **One** answer is required for each question. Each option can be used once, more than once or not at all.

 A 14-year-old boy, who usually vomits after having treatment with chemotherapy, starts to become nauseous upon entering the treatment room.

 A 5-year-old girl, who is given ice cream bought from the hospital shop before her chemotherapy, starts to feel nauseous not only when given the ice cream, but now also when she sees the shop.

 A 10-year-old boy, who became frightened of his next-door neighbour's white poodle after it repeatedly chased him around the garden while barking, is now too frightened to approach any dog.

(Q168) Remembering to buy flowers for your partner as he always subsequently becomes more affectionate.

(Q169) Avoiding your flat as you frequently fight with your flatmates.

(Q170) The payouts associated with slot machines.

(Q171) Training a dog to fetch the mail by leaving dog biscuits closer and closer to the door every morning.

(Q172) Not buying your girlfriend chocolates for her birthday as she always becomes angry at being given a calorific gift.

(Q173) A factory worker being paid £5 per pair of trousers sewn.

EMI 8

Options:

A Acute schizophrenia-like psychotic episode
B Delirium
C Dementia in Alzheimer's disease
D Depressive disorder
E Dissociative fugue
F Encephalitis
G Korsakoff's syndrome
H Transient global amnesia
I Transient ischaemic attack
J Vascular dementia
K Wernicke's encephalopathy

For each of the following scenarios, choose the **most appropriate disease/disorder** from the list above. Each question requires **one** answer only. Each option can be used once, more than once or not at all.

 A 74-year-old woman on a surgical ward became generally confused and, thinking that she was at home, started to mistake the night staff for her relatives. When reassured, she became irritable and angry.

 A 72-year-old woman on a psychiatric ward complained of forgetfulness and word-finding difficulties. On testing, her memory was impaired for recent and remote events equally, but her performance improved with encouragement.

 A 70-year-old writer was noted to have become increasingly forgetful, with difficulties in naming and word finding. On testing, her memory for remote events was unaffected, although her memory for recent events was impaired.

A 68-year-old hypertensive woman, after hearing about her son's death, suddenly became forgetful and was unable to register any new information. She drove to Scotland but did not lose her personal identity.

 An 18-year-old university student complained of a severe progressive headache for a few hours and then experienced a seizure before starting to display odd behaviour. She appeared drowsy and was talking to herself. She also had impaired comprehension.

EMI 9

Options:

A   Anterior parietal lobe lesion
B   Dominant parietal lobe lesion
C   Dominant temporal lobe lesion
D   Frontal lobe lesion
E   Gerstmann's syndrome
F   Lesion in deep midline structures
G   Non-dominant parietal lobe lesion
H   Non-dominant temporal lobe lesion
I   Occipital lobe lesion
J   Posterior parietal lobe lesion

For each of the following, choose the **most appropriate** option from the list above. Each question requires **one** answer only. Each option can be used once, more than once or not at all.

 Q179   Prosopagnosia and alexia without agraphia.

 Q180   Amnesic syndrome and hypersomnia.

 Q181   Disinhibition, impulsive behaviour and aggressive outbursts.

Q182   Primary motor aphasia.

Q183   Primary sensory aphasia.

 Q184   Hemisomatognosia and anosognosia.

EMI 10

Options:

A   Confabulation
B   Dyscalculia
C   Hyperorality
D   Hyperphagia
E   Hypersalivation
F   Hypersexuality
G   Hypersomnia
H   Impotence
I   Simultanagnosia
J   Visual hallucinations

For each of the following syndromes, choose the **most character-istic** symptom(s). The number of answers required for each syndrome is indicated in parentheses. Each option may be used once, more than once or not at all.

(Q185)   Kluver–Bucy syndrome.   (2)

(Q186)   Korsakoff's syndrome.   (1)

(Q187)   Gerstmann's syndrome.   (1)

(Q188)   Balint's syndrome.   (1)

(Q189)   Prader–Willi syndrome.   (1)

(Q190)   Charles Bonnet syndrome.   (1)

(Q191)   Kleine–Levin syndrome.   (4)

Paper 1:
Answers

(A1) **True.** Perceptual set was defined by Allport in 1955. It is a tendency to perceive some aspects of data and ignore others. (1: p.220)

(A2) **True.** They are based on population studies and describe all personalities as either belonging to discrete categories (type theories) or posit that human variation may be described using a limited number of continuous qualities common to the whole population (trait theories). (2: p.88)

(A3) **False.** The halo effect occurs when a person's positive or negative traits seem to 'spill over' from one area of their personality. It allows us to guess what people are like when we have only very limited information about them. (1: p.332)

(A4) **False.** It is increased by similarity in attitudes, proximity, exposure (geographical), familiarity, physical attractiveness, complementarity of resources, perceived competence and reciprocal liking. It allows initiation of relationships. (1: p.401)

(A5) **True.** (1: p.411)

(A6) **True.** He will also try to re-define the situation and diffuse responsibility in order to justify not intervening. (1: p.435)

(A7) **False.** The effects of TV violence are arousal, disinhibition, imitation and desensitisation. (1: p.516)

(A8) **False.** Conformity increases with group number and perceived social status of members. (1: p.387)

(A9) **True.** Milgram demonstrated that individuals will obey instructions (even those against their beliefs) when they are in certain situations. Participants were instructed by an experimenter to deliver electric shocks to stooges. They were ordered to increase the voltage, but despite the stooges screaming as if in pain, 75% of the participants continued to deliver shocks. The experimenter is perceived as an authority; individuals believe that they have no choice and can therefore deny responsibility for their actions. On the basis of this experiment it is thought that obedience is increased with distance from stooges and the presence of the instructor. (1: p.392)

(A10) **True.** Also subtests of verbal, visual, abstract and quantitative reasoning. (3: p.41)

(A11) **True.** The other performance subtests are object assembly, picture arrangement, picture completion and digit symbol. (4: p.110)

(A12) **False.** Fluid intelligence includes untaught abilities such as problem-solving, whereas crystallised intelligence is defined as a cumulative, learned and experience-based acquired knowledge. (2: p.83)

(A13) **True.** According to the theory of fundamental attribution error, we tend to believe that personal factors are responsible for the behaviour of others, rather than their situation (situational factors). (1: p.345)

(A14) **False.** Kohlberg formulated this theory. The three levels in ascending order are preconventional (punishment and reward orientation – up to age 7 years), conventional (good boy/good girl and authority orientation – ages 7–13 years) and postconventional morality (social contract and ethical principle orientation). Kohlberg estimated that less than 10% of his adult subjects showed stage 6 reasoning. Before he died, he eliminated stage 6 from his theory. Level 3 is now referred to as high-stage principled reasoning. (5: p.33) (6: p.85)

(A15) **False.** This is assimilation. Accommodation refers to the modification of existing schemas in order to comprehend new information. (3: p.50)

(A16) **False.** Authoritative parenting involves nurturing parents with high expectations and strict rules. Other forms of parenting styles are the permissive (unconditionally nurturing) and authoritarian–restrictive (controlling and less nurturing) styles. (3: p.48)

(A17) **False.** Gender constancy (consistency) is when the child realises that gender is unchangeable. This usually occurs between the ages of 6 and 7 years. (7: p.72)

(A18) **True.** (7: p.74)

(A19) **True.** These are features of long-term memory. Furthermore, there is little or no decline in sensory or working memory with age. (7: p.79)

(A20) **False.** Between 8 months and 1 year of age. (7: p.70)

(A21) **False.** They are more likely to do so. Other sequelae to childhood physical abuse include aggression, neurological/cognitive impairments and developmental delay. (3: p.49)

(A22) **False.** It requires several trials. It is insight learning (a type of cognitive learning) that is learned suddenly after one trial. (5: pp.1, 2, 5)

(A23) **True.** (5: p.2)

(A24) **False.** Figure ground differentiation, brightness discrimination, fixing, scanning and tracking are believed to be innate. Perceptual constancy and depth recognition are learned. (5: p.14)

(A25) **True.** Attending to two sources of information simultaneously is known as divided attention. (5: p.16)

(A26) **False.** It is around 5%. This is more commonly known as a photographic memory. (5: p.17)

(A27) **True.** Storage capacity is 7 ± 2. When working memory is full, new items are added by displacing old ones. (5: p.17)

(A28) **False.** This is retroactive interference. Proactive interference refers to previously learned information impairing new learning. (5: p.22)

(A29) **True.** It describes the relationship between arousal and performance; both high and low arousal lead to impaired performance. (5: p.40)

(A30) **True.** Thereby also increasing penetration of larger antibiotic molecules. (2: p.609)

(A31) **False.** It increases permeability for 24 hours. (2: p.608)

(A32) **True.** As are diazepam, chlorpromazine and amitriptyline. (2: p.609)

(A33) **True.** (2: p.611)

(A34) **True.** Initially it is eliminated by first-order kinetics; at higher doses it follows zero-order kinetics. (2: p.611)

(A35) **True.** As it is a hepatic enzyme inhibitor. (2: p.611)

(A36) **False.** It is affected by their increased body fat. They also have less body water and albumin than younger adults. This leads to an increased volume of distribution, a longer duration of action for some fat-soluble drugs (e.g. diazepam) and a reduction in the amount of drugs bound to albumins (therefore more of the active free drug is available, such as occurs with warfarin or phenytoin). (8: p.230)

(A37) **True.** Other side-effects include nausea, vomiting, ataxia, agitation (especially in the elderly), leucopenia, paraesthesia and the Stevens–Johnson syndrome. (9)

(A38) **False.** It commonly causes them. Other adverse effects include drowsiness, insomnia, depression and (more rarely) agitation. (9)

(A39) **True.** Particularly dystonic reactions and akathisia. (9)

(A40) **True.** Other adverse effects include neutropenia, potentially fatal agranulocytosis, hypersalivation, dry mouth, agitation, hepatitis, pericarditis, myocarditis and elevated plasma CK concentration. (9)

(A41) **False.** It may cause it at toxic doses. Other signs of lithium intoxication include increasing GI and CNS disturbances; withdrawal of treatment is required. (9)

(A42) **True.** Hence it is likely to be safer in overdose than traditional TCAs. (10: p.679)

(A43) **True.** Depressed ST segments and flattened T waves may also occur. (10: p.679)

(A44) **False.** In overdose, heart rate may be increased or decreased depending partly on the degree of conduction disturbance. (10: p.679)

(A45) **True.** As are postural hypotension, confusion, increased salivation, GI disturbances and sexual dysfunction. (9)

(A46) **False.** Rarely. (9)

(A47) **True.** Receptors D1,5 increase and D2,3,4 decrease adenylate cyclase activity. (3: p.165) (11: p.312)

(A48) **False.** As GABA aminotransferase inhibits GABA metabolism, GABA breakdown is prevented. (3: p.185)

(A49) **True.** By glutaminase. (11: p.387)

(A50) **False.** It has little affinity for these or for histaminergic receptors. (11: p.246)

(A51) **True.** And therefore it is the TCA of choice in the treatment of OCD. (10: p.678)

(A52) **False.** It is a NARI (noradrenaline (norepinephrine) reuptake inhibitor). It has little affinity for cholinergic or histaminergic receptors. (11: p.235)

(A53) **False.** It is DOPAC and HVA (homovanillic acid) that are breakdown products of dopamine. VMA (vanillyl mandelic acid) is a breakdown product of norepinephrine. (3: pp.154–5)

(A54) **True.** As well as serotonin and GABA activity. It is thought to decrease central acetylcholine activity. (5: p.257)

(A55) **True.** Other drugs that induce liver enzymes include barbiturates, alcohol, phenobarbitone, phenytoin, primidone, rifampicin and cigarette smoking. (3: p.186) (11: p.211)

(A56) **True.** (12: pp.39, 40, 47)

(A57) **False.** This is the term used for a placebo that contains a pharmaceutical drug; it is usually used to reduce failure of blinding in randomised controlled trials (as clinicians might be able to guess which subjects are on active treatment if they develop adverse effects). (12: pp.39, 40, 47)

(A58) **False.** Characteristically in organic disorders, although it can be a symptom of catatonia. (13: p.157) (14)

(A59) **True.** It lasts for almost 25 hours. (13: p.80)

(A60) **False.** 10% of non-schizophrenic patients experience FRS. Furthermore, 20% of people with schizophrenia do not have FRS. (2: p.265)

(A61) **False.** It is characterised by negative symptoms such as flattening of affect, poverty of speech and loss of motivation. Type I describes acute schizophrenia with hallucinations, delusions and thought disorder. There is a better response to antipsychotic medication in type I compared with type II. (13: p.163)

(A62) **True.** Such as in states of fatigue, sleep deprivation or sensory deprivation. It also occurs in adults. (13: p.232)

(A63) **True.** It occurs in 25–30% of cases. It sometimes occurs after the use of alcohol and drugs (especially LSD, cannabis and TCAs). (13: p.237)

(A64) **True.** It is also a symptom of bulbar palsy. Pseudobulbar palsy results from a UMN lesion. The dysarthria of pseudo-bulbar palsy is described as 'Donald Duck' speech; the tongue is small and contracted, palatal movements are absent, the jaw jerk is exaggerated and there may be emotional lability. Bulbar palsy occurs in LMN lesions. The speech has a nasal twang, and wasting of the muscles of the tongue is seen. (15: p.16)

(A65) **False.** It means speaking in a private language. It can occur in schizophrenia, but more often in normal people. (13: p.175)

(A66) **False.** Individuals are able to speak, understand speech and write, but cannot read with understanding (alexia). It is an agnosic alexia without dysgraphia. (13: p.176)

(A67) **True.** They may also occur as fears or ruminations. Compulsions, in comparison, may be rituals or acts. (13: p.338)

(A68) **False.** Obsessional symptoms are always recognised as one's own. (13: p.338)

(A69) **True.** Distractibility may result in meals being interrupted. (13: p.348)

(A70) **True.** The Pickwickian syndrome is also known as obstructive sleep apnoea. (13: p.345)

(A71) **True.** Paranoid personality disorder is characterised by hostility, distrust, suspiciousness, quarrelsomeness and quickness to take offence. Individuals go to enormous lengths to defend their rights and beliefs. (13: p.382)

(A72) **False.** Married people in general are healthier, live longer and suffer less mental illness. However, there can be a high incidence of mental distress at the time of deciding to get married. (7: p.74)

(A73) **False.** Integrity versus Despair is the last stage of Erikson's theory of psychosocial development. In early adulthood the conflicts encountered are Intimacy versus Isolation. Fulfilment and commitment are considered to be successful outcomes at these stages, respectively. (3: p.43) (7: p.73)

(A74) **False.** Within 6–12 months. (3: p.58)

(A75) **True.** Primary delusions do not occur in response to other psychopathological phenomena such as low mood. There are four types, namely autochthonous delusions, delusional perception, delusional atmosphere and delusional memory. (13: p.120)

(A76) **False.** This is Capgras syndrome. In Cotard's syndrome there are nihilistic and hypochondriacal delusions. (13: p.137)

(A77) **False.** This is true in folie imposée. In folie communiqué, the beliefs are maintained despite separation. The other two types of communicated insanity are folie induite, when a psychotic person adds the delusions of another on to their own, and folie simultanée, when two or more people become psychotic simultaneously. (13: p.140)

(A78) **True.** Distortion of shape (i.e. micropsia, macropsia and dysmegalopsia) has been described in parietal lobe lesions. (13: p.94)

(A79) **True.** This is said to occur when perceptions in different modalities, although coming from the same source, appear to be separate and sometimes in conflict (e.g. visual and auditory percepts from the television). It can also occur in organic states. (13: p.95)

(A80) **False.** These occur when an incomplete percept is altered and 'filled in' by the mind's eye, so that it becomes meaningful. They occur with inattention and are banished by attention. (13: p.96)

(A81) **True.** These are abnormal perceptions of miniature things – usually little animals or men. Individuals often have insight. (13: p.105)

(A82) **False.** Depression. They are also known to occur in epilepsy in addition to other neurological and psychiatric conditions. An autoscopic hallucination ('phantom mirror image') is a rare perceptual experience in which one sees a hallucination of oneself. For a hallucination to qualify as autoscopic, it must be in the visual, kinaesthetic and somatic modalities. (13: p.106)

(A83) **True.** Often with beliefs of control. (13: p.107)

(A84) **True.** (13: p.127)

(A85) **True.** This transformation would be precipitated by the occurrence of a significant major event. (13: p.129)

(A86) **True.** And lower for depression and suicidal ideation. (13: p.131)

(A87) **False.** Sleep drunkenness is when the normal process of waking rapidly is slowed down, resulting in a feeling of drowsiness and incompetence for a prolonged period of time after waking. (13: p.57)

(A88) **True.** This is a very rare syndrome, usually occurring in young men, in which attacks of somnolence and megaphagia (voracious eating) occur. (13: p.57)

(A89) **True.** And also when relaxed (e.g. dreaming) or fooled (e.g. by jokes). (5: p.160)

(A90) **False.** It is the day residue, not night residue, and refers to memories of the day; nocturnal stimuli refer to both internal and external stimuli (e.g. pain and noise). (5: p.162)

(A91) **False.** This is the 'female Oedipal complex', and as such is a phenomenon of the phallic stage. (5: p.164)

(A92) **True.** Archetypes are myths common to all cultures (i.e. universal) and are contained within the collective unconscious. The Anima refers to the female elements within a man, and the Shadow refers to one's animal instincts. Other archetypes include the Animus (male elements in a woman), the Persona (which masks an individual's personality), the Self (a central archetype holding unacknowledged aspects of the self), the Great Mother, the Wise Old Man and the Hero. (16: p.100)

(A93) **False.** It starts to develop at 6 months. Prior to this the baby occupies the paranoid–schizoid position. (5: p.167)

(A94) **True.** This was created by Moreno and has been integrated not only into creative occupational therapy activities but also into both gestalt and family therapy. (16: p.179)

(A95) **True.** The '*I and thou*' principle encourages individuals to talk to, rather than at, others. '*No gossiping*' refers to addressing others directly rather than talking about them as if they were absent. Other principles include '*I language*' (when referring to parts of one's body, the 'it' needs to be changed to 'I', e.g. 'my legs are tired' becomes 'I am tired'), *'dialogue'* (where the individual creates a conversation between two split parts of him- or herself), *'making the rounds'* (addressing each individual instead of remarking on the group as a whole), *'unfinished business'* (addressing unresolved feelings from the past), *'exaggeration'* (acting out unwanted feelings in an exaggerated fashion) and *'reversal'* (acting out the opposite of unwanted feelings). (16: p.180)

(A96) **True.** (16: p.175)

(A97) **True.** (13: pp.241–68)

(A98) **False.** It is described by schizophrenic patients and may occur as the first symptom. (13: pp.241–68)

(A99) **True.** Gender identity is an individual's perception and self-awareness with respect to gender. (13: p.272)

(A100) **False.** The difference is clearly established before puberty. (13: p.274)

(A101) **True.** There is often extreme social disapproval of paedophilia, with perpetrators experiencing feelings of rejection and severe depressive reactions. Suicide is not uncommon. (13: p.278)

(A102) **True.** 50% of suicides occur in the first 3 months of imprisonment, the majority by hanging, and 50% of inmates have a history of deliberate self-harm. (17: p.152)

(A103) **True.** They have also been found to have decreased numbers of 5HT receptors in the frontal cortex and hippocampus. (17: p.152)

(A104) **True.** Depression is most likely to occur in the first trimester, and is associated with a previous history of depression, marital conflict and anxiety about the baby. Depression in the last trimester may progress into the puerperium. (17: p.378)

(A105) **False.** The correct figure is 10%. Symptoms include irritability, tearfulness, tiredness, anxiety about not being able to care for the baby, and poor libido, sleep, concentration and appetite. (17: p.380)

(A106) **False.** It is sodium valproate or carbamazepine. (17: p.60)

(A107) **True.** Also where the illness shows an irregular pattern. (8: p.93)

(A108) **False.** They have identified it in up to 30% of male and 10% of female admissions. (10: p.541)

(A109) **True.** It is also higher among chefs, barmen, brewery workers, executive salesmen, seamen, journalists and doctors. (10: p.543)

(A110) **False.** These are features of Korsakoff's syndrome. Characteristic features of Wernicke's encephalopathy are ataxia and ophthalmoplegia, with nystagmus and impaired consciousness. Peripheral neuropathy may also be present. (5: p.343)

(A111) **True.** He also suggested that pyknic build is associated with cyclothymic personality types, and asthenic build with schizotypal personality types. (10: p.159)

(A112) **False.** The reverse is true. The total prevalence of personality disorders ranges from 6% to 15%. Among psychiatry outpatients and inpatients a prevalence of up to 50% has been reported. (10: pp.173–4)

(A113) **False.** They are classified with organic mental disorders. (10: p.162)

(A114) **True.** Others include anaemia, chronic infection, diabetes, hypothyroidism and carcinomas. (10: p.478)

A115 **True.** These are acute psychotic disorders (i.e. with onset within 2 weeks), in which the hallucinations, delusions and emotional state of the patient are constantly changing (even within the same day). However, should schizophrenic symptoms persist for more than 1 month, the diagnosis should be changed to one of schizophrenia. (14: p.102)

A116 **False.** This describes bipolar II. Bipolar I is characterised by the occurrence of one or more manic episodes (although individuals often also experience major depressive episodes). (18: pp.350–9)

A117 **True.** According to DSM-IV, atypical depression is characterised by preserved mood reactivity and two or more of the following: increased appetite, weight or sleep, leaden paralysis (a heavy leaden feeling in the limbs) or a longstanding pattern of interpersonal rejection sensitivity. (18: p.386)

A118 **True.** As is the presence of retardation and delusions. (19: p.893)

A119 **False.** It is variable, chronic and fluctuating. (14: p.140)

A120 **True.** Symptoms resolve rapidly once the stressor is removed. (14: p.147)

A121 **True.** Particularly if their onset is associated with a traumatic life event. However, more intractable states can develop in the presence of insoluble problems or interpersonal difficulties. Those lasting for 1–2 years are often resistant to treatment. (14: p.152)

A122 **True.** Other common causes include vascular disease, head injury, tumours, infections and occasionally dementia. (20: p.965)

A123 **True.** (20: p.966)

A124 **True.** (20: p.966)

(A125) **False.** Agraphia is the inability to write. Agraphaesthesia is the inability to recognise figures (letters or numbers) drawn on the hand (with the eyes closed). (20: p.968)

(A126) **False.** In terms of speech dominance and handedness: 95% of right-handers are left hemisphere dominant and 5% are right hemisphere dominant; 70% of left-handers are left hemisphere dominant, 15% are right hemisphere dominant and 15% are bilateral. The Annett Handedness Questionnaire is commonly used to determine handedness. (20: p.974)

(A127) **True.** Although prominent and vivid, they are silent and non-threatening, unlike those in psychiatric disease or drug-induced states. (10: p.406)

(A128) **False.** (10: p.407)

(A129) **True.** Methadone, like all opiates, causes suppression of the cough reflex, constipation and respiratory depression. Pupillary constriction does occur, but is less marked than with morphine. However, the withdrawal syndrome is similar to that for morphine. (10: p.567)

(A130) **True.** As is anxiety. Depression is also a risk factor for increased morbidity and mortality following myocardial infarction. (10: p.461)

(A131) **False.** The reverse is true. (10: p.464)

(A132) **False.** It is associated with impaired sexual functioning. (10: p.477)

(A133) **True.** Genetic linkage has been suggested. (10: p.177)

EMI 1

(A134) E. Other symptoms include clouding of consciousness, ataxia, ophthalmoplegia and peripheral neuropathy. (5: p.342)

(A135) D, H. Meningococcal meningitis. (21: p.368)

(A136) B. (10: p.406) (21: p.230)

(A137) I. Other symptoms include bradykinesia, bradyphrenia (slowness in comprehension and response), micrographia, lead pipe and cogwheel rigidity, postural changes, a festinant gait with poor arm swing, dribbling, dysphagia and monotonous speech progressing to slurred dysarthria. There is no sensory loss. (22: p.1182)

EMI 2

(A138) E, I. (9)

(A139) A, B. (9)

(A140) D, J. (9)

(A141) C, G. This is an especially dangerous combination. Clomipramine should only be started 3 weeks after MAOI treatment has been stopped. (9)

EMI 3

(A142) C. It has subscales for somatic symptoms, anxiety, insomnia, depression and social functioning. (10: p.68)

(A143) E. (10: p.68)

(A144) F. (10: p.68)

(A145) A. (10: p.68)

(A146) D. (4: p.121)

EMI 4

(A147) **F.** Trazodone rarely causes priapism (this is an indication to discontinue treatment immediately). It has fewer antimuscarinic and cardiovascular effects than amitriptyline. (9)

(A148) **C.** Mianserin may cause leucopenia, agranulocytosis and aplastic anaemia (especially in the elderly). FBC monitoring is important; treatment should be stopped and an FBC repeated if any signs or symptoms of infection are reported. (9)

(A149) **B.** Lofepramine is a non-sedating tricyclic compound. Unlike conventional TCAs it is not cardiotoxic in overdose. Hence it is likely to be safer, although caution is still recommended. (10: p.679)

(A150) **E.** Although reboxetine is structurally related to fluoxetine, it belongs to the class of NARIs (selective norepinephrine reuptake inhibitors) and has no significant effect on other neurotransmitters. (10: p.693)

(A151) **A.** Clomipramine is a tricyclic compound. It can also be used in the adjunctive treatment of cataplexy associated with narcolepsy. (9)

EMI 5

(A152) **A.** Attachment refers to the tendency to remain close to certain individuals (attachment figures). (5: p.64)

(A153) **C.** This is Erikson's final stage of psychosocial development, which occurs in old age. (5: p.467)

(A154) **G.** Transitional or comfort objects may help to relieve the anxiety felt on separation, and can include objects such as teddy bears, or even religion or music. They are chosen between the ages of 4 and 18 months. Adults can also benefit from their use (e.g. in cases of divorce or bereavement). (5: p.168)

(A155) **D.** (5: p.72)

(A156) **E.** The permissive (laissez-faire), authoritative and authoritarian approaches. (7: p.59)

(A157) **B.** The easy child is sociable, easygoing and predictable; the difficult child cries a lot and is active, unpredictable and socially inhibited. The temperament of the slow to warm up child lies between these two. (7: p.61)

(A158) **H.** This occurs between the ages of 2 and 7 years. It is during this stage that precausal logic, animism and authoritarian morality occur. (3: p.51)

EMI 6

(A159) **D.** By 2 years of age, children have a vocabulary of approximately 300 words. Between 18 months and 3 years their speech is telegraphic (the 'two-word phrase' stage). (7: p.64)

(A160) **I.** (7: p.65)

(A161) **H.** This is knowing about the existence of objects that are out of sight. (7: p.62)

(A162) **G.** The pre-operational stage was described as occurring between the ages of 2 and 7 years. Egocentrism, animism and centration (focusing on a single quality at a time) are all features of this stage. (7: p.63)

(A163) **G.** Egocentrism is the inability to view from the perspective of others. Conservation is the understanding that the amount of a substance remains the same even when the form is changed (e.g. by pouring water from a tall to a short glass). Children are also unable to understand transductive reasoning, seriation and execute operations during this stage of their development. (7: p.63) (6: p.77)

(A164) **F.** (7: p.65)

EMI 7

(A165) **I.** This is classical conditioning. Chemotherapy is the UCS, nausea is the UCR, and the treatment room becomes the CS. After a number of chemotherapy sessions (i.e. 'trials'), the repeated pairing of chemotherapy with the treatment room leads the teenager to associate these together, therefore inducing nausea even before treatment starts (the CR). (6: p.237)

(A166) **J.** The chemotherapy is the UCS, ice cream is the CS, and nausea is the CR. However, now the ice cream acts as a UCS and the shop becomes the CS. This process is known as higher-order conditioning (i.e. second order if there is only a second CS, third order if there is a third CS, etc.). In general, the higher the order the weaker the conditioning. (6: p.237) (5: p.2)

(A167) **D.** Generalisation is when the CR (fear) of a given stimulus (the poodle) can now be elicited by other similar stimuli (all dogs). (5: p.2)

(A168) **G.** The behaviour 'buying flowers' increases as a result of a rewarding stimulus, namely the affectionate behaviour. Positive reinforcement increases a behaviour by giving a positive stimulus (i.e. reward). (5: pp.5–6) (6: p.243)

F. The behaviour 'avoiding your flat' is increased by removal of an aversive stimulus (fighting with your flatmates). Negative reinforcement increases a behaviour by removing an aversive stimulus. (5: pp.5–6) (6: p.243)

 M. On this type of schedule, reinforcement (pay off) occurs only after a certain number of responses (plays) have been made, but that number varies unpredictably (the player has no way of predicting when the payout will occur). (6: p.247)

 K. Shaping is a technique used in people with learning disability, where successively closer approximations to the desired behaviour are reinforced until it is finally achieved. Chaining, on the other hand, is where a complex behaviour is first broken down into steps, which are taught separately and, when achieved, finally linked together to produce the complex behaviour. Forward chaining refers to learning the first steps of the behaviour initially. Backward chaining refers to learning the last steps initially. (5: pp.7–8)

 H. The behaviour 'buying chocolates' is decreased as a result of an aversive stimulus, namely 'anger'. Punishment decreases the probability of an event by delivery of an aversive stimulus. (6: p.243)

 C. On this type of schedule, reinforcement (payment) depends on the number of responses made (number of pairs of trousers sewn). (6: p.247)

EMI 8

 B. Disorientation and labile mood of sudden onset in an elderly medical inpatient suggest delirium. (20: pp.993–6)

 D. In contrast, in dementia, subjective reporting of complaints is uncommon, remote memory is not usually impaired until late, and performance is unaffected by encouragement. (20: pp.1015–16)

(A176) **C.** This is a typical description of dementia.

(A177) **H.** Although the son's death was a stressful event, not losing identity differentiates this from fugue. Sudden onset of memory loss for recent events, an inability to register new impressions and retrograde amnesia are clinical hallmarks of transient global amnesia. (20: p.1058)

(A178) **F.** Encephalitis usually presents with severe progressive headache, vomiting, papilloedema, reduced level of consciousness and coma; other features include delirium, seizures and psychotic symptoms. Focal neurological signs and symptoms of temporal lobe syndrome (dysphasia, auditory hallucinations and bizarre behaviour) are most suggestive of herpes simplex encephalitis. (20: p.1066)

EMI 9

Reference for all (20: pp.964–9)

(A179) **I.**

(A180) **F.**

(A181) **D.**

(A182) **D.**

(A183) **C.**

(A184) **G.**

EMI 10

(A185) **C, F.** Kluver–Bucy syndrome (also characterised by visual agnosia and loss of fear) can occur as part of Pick's disease, Alzheimer's dementia, arteriosclerosis, cerebral tumours and herpes simplex encephalitis. (2: pp.18, 379)

(A186) **A.** This is characterised by prominent impairment of recent memory and difficulty learning new material with preservation of immediate recall and procedural memory. Confabulation is not a prerequisite for diagnosis. (2: p.425) (14)

(A187) **B.** (2: p.19)

(A188) **I.** This occurs in bilateral lesions of the occipital lobe. It includes optic ataxia (abnormal visual guidance of limb movements), oculomotor apraxia (inability to visually scan the environment) and simultanagnosia (inability to see more than one object at a time). (3: p.97)

(A189) **D.** Prader–Willi syndrome is a chromosomal disorder caused by a partial deletion on the long arm of chromosome 15. Symptoms include severe congenital hypotonia, and feeding difficulties with poor weight gain up to the age of 2 years, followed by mild mental retardation, short stature, hypogonadism, a voracious appetite and obesity. (3: p.204) (23: p.302)

(A190) **J.** In this syndrome, visual hallucinations that are vivid and well formed occur in clear consciousness, and insight is preserved. They can persist for seconds or hours at a time, and usually occur in the elderly. The aetiology is unknown. (4: p.295)

(A191) **C, D, F, G.** (2: p.399)

Paper 2:
Questions

Q1 In Maslow's hierarchy of needs, the needs lower down the hierarchy must be satisfied before the needs higher up can be attended to.

Q2 Adding new cognitions increases cognitive dissonance.

Q3 The fundamental attribution error refers to the tendency to favour situational rather than personal factors in appraising human behaviour.

Q4 Pluralistic ignorance will negatively influence the likelihood of intervention by a bystander in an emergency.

Q5 Research shows that watching violence on television results in vicarious catharsis.

Q6 According to the hydraulic model of instinct, aggression is spontaneous rather than reactive, and does not occur in response to environmental stimuli.

Q7 The Thurstone scale is an 11-point scale for measuring arousal.

Q8 According to Lewin, in autocratic leaderships interaction with the leader is task related.

Q9 The Intelligence Quotient is expressed as a ratio of chronological age over mental age and multiplied by 100.

Q10 Similarities is a verbal subtest of the WAIS.

(Q11) The National Adult Reading Test is designed to check premorbid intelligence.

(Q12) Personal construct theory is an example of an idiographic theory of personality.

(Q13) Hemisomatognosia may be a symptom of non-dominant temporal lobe damage.

(Q14) Niharika suggested the term 'schizoid' and believed that this type of personality is related to schizophrenia.

(Q15) Lorenz explained attachment as a form of imprinting.

(Q16) Precausal logic was described as a feature of the pre-operational stage by Kohlberg.

(Q17) Language development is usually slower in boys than in girls.

(Q18) Up to 40% of all children below the age of 5 years have an imaginary friend.

(Q19) Ethnic identity is more easily achieved in the absence of actual discrimination.

(Q20) Homosexuality is more likely to develop following sexual abuse in childhood.

(Q21) Kohlberg defined both reward and authority orientations as part of the conventional stage in his theory of moral development.

(Q22) Cognitive learning is a form of associative learning.

(Q23) Money can act as a secondary reinforcer.

(Q24) Accommodation develops at 2 months of age and colour vision develops at 4 months.

Q25   The habituation method is a way of studying the development of perceptual constancy in infants.

Q26   LTM is not required to help to chunk information into working memory.

Q27   Children have a total amnesia for events before 3 years of age.

Q28   Episodic and semantic memories are types of explicit memory.

Q29   Maslow's hierarchy of needs incorporates aspects of both extrinsic and intrinsic theories of motivation.

Q30   Displacement and secondary elaboration are processes involved in changing the latent into the manifest dream.

Q31   Freud's structural model, consisting of the unconscious, preconscious and conscious, pre-dates the topographical model.

Q32   According to Freud, the anal stage of psychosexual development occurs from 18 months to 5 years.

Q33   Feeling, intuition, sensation and believing are the four operations of the mind, according to Jungian theorists.

Q34   According to Klein, a child introjects objects believed to be good.

Q35   Gestalt therapy is usually practised on a one-to-one basis.

Q36   Concepts of cognitive analytic therapy include turns and snags.

Q37   Interpersonal therapy is unstructured and involves a limited number of sessions.

(Q38) Drugs with anticholinergic activity increase absorption from the small bowel.

(Q39) At peak plasma concentrations, the rate of drug absorption equals the rate of elimination.

(Q40) First-pass metabolism of a drug takes place in the hepatic portal system.

(Q41) Tranylcypromine inhibits hepatic metabolism.

(Q42) St John's wort reduces the efficacy of the oral contraceptive pill.

(Q43) Lamotrigine induces cytochrome P450.

(Q44) Phenelzine has been associated with fatal progressive hepatocellular necrosis.

(Q45) Lofepramine is more sedating than amitriptyline.

(Q46) Alopecia has been reported with fluoxetine use.

(Q47) Diazepam may occasionally cause urinary retention.

(Q48) Pimozide is more sedating than chlorpromazine.

(Q49) Olanzapine is commonly associated with blood dyscrasias.

(Q50) Clozapine is known to cause hypersalivation, but not dry mouth.

(Q51) Olanzapine rarely causes photosensitivity and an elevated CK concentration.

(Q52) Hyperprolactinaemia is a known side-effect of risperidone, but not olanzapine.

(Q53) Quetiapine may cause elevation of the plasma thyroid hormone concentration.

Q54   Shortening of the QT interval has been reported with amisulpride.

Q55   GABA is metabolised by GABA aminotransferase.

Q56   The NMDA glutamate receptor is associated with a calcium channel.

Q57 MAO_B is reversibly inhibited by moclobemide.

Q58   Blockade of alpha$_1$ receptors by antipsychotics can result in postural hypotension and ejaculatory failure.

Q59   Venlafaxine inhibits both 5HT and norepinephrine reuptake at the postsynaptic terminal.

Q60   Tryptophan is a precursor of 5HT.

Q61   MHPG and VMA are breakdown products of norepinephrine.

Q62   Buprenorphine, a partial agonist at the mu receptor, is used as maintenance treatment in cases of heroin addiction.

Q63   ECT results in down-regulation of beta receptors.

Q64   The beneficial effect seen in patients by simply providing attention is termed the Hawthorne effect.

Q65   The term reciprocation is used when two effective treatments given together produce no greater effect than either given alone.

Q66   Age disorientation can be a symptom of schizophrenia.

Q67   Dereistic thinking is a common feature of schizophrenia.

Q68   Over-inclusive thinking occurs in obsessional personalities.

(Q69) Made experiences are delusions of control.

(Q70) Depersonalisation is an experience that may last from seconds to hours.

(Q71) Dysphonia is the loss of ability to vocalise.

(Q72) Echolalia is a symptom of catatonia.

(Q73) A patient with pure word blindness cannot name colours despite being able to perceive them.

(Q74) The sense of passage of time is disturbed in ecstasy states.

(Q75) With regard to the stages of bereavement, disorganisation precedes preoccupation.

(Q76) Panic disorder has been established as a separate diagnostic category in ICD-10 but not DSM-IV.

(Q77) In OCD, individuals know that the obsessional thoughts are their own.

(Q78) Obsessional symptoms may occur in schizophrenia, where they usually have a bizarre character.

(Q79) Phobias are unreasonable and appropriate fears.

(Q80) In histrionic personality disorder, impulsive acts are usually aggressive.

(Q81) The mental illness most consistently associated with an increased risk of violent behaviour is borderline personality disorder.

(Q82) Individuals with paranoid personality disorder frequently have obsessional ideas.

Q83 Patients with emotionally unstable PD (impulsive type) are impulsive and irritable most of the time.

Q84 Anankasts find the initiation or completion of any activity difficult.

Q85 In dependent PD there is a preoccupation with criticism and a fear of rejection by others.

Q86 Autochthonous delusions, also known as Wahneinfall, are the same as delusional intuition.

Q87 Thought block is a first-rank symptom.

Q88 Delusional atmosphere is experienced as unpleasant.

Q89 Ekbom's syndrome is exclusively a delusional illness.

Q90 Pareidolia is a normal phenomenon.

Q91 Visual and auditory hallucinations occurring simultaneously are suggestive of temporal lobe epilepsy.

Q92 Illusions are transformations of perceptions.

Q93 Olfactory hallucinations commonly form the aura in temporal lobe epilepsy.

Q94 Hypnopompic hallucinations are normal phenomena that occur while going to sleep.

Q95 Reflex hallucinations are the hallucinatory form of synaesthesia.

Q96 Persecutory delusions may function to protect self-esteem.

Q97 Sleep paralysis is an inability to move when between waking and sleep.

Q98   In jamais vu, a familiar event feels as if it has never been experienced before.

Q99   Marked suggestibility is a prominent feature in confabulation.

Q100   The Ganser syndrome is a type of dissociative disorder.

Q101   Body dysmorphic disorder and transsexualism usually take the psychopathological form of an overvalued idea.

Q102   Gender identity is developed on the basis of gender role.

Q103   Paedophilia is included in the disorders of sexual preference in ICD-10.

Q104   Exhibitionism is the commonest type of sexual offence.

Q105   PTSD is a risk factor for suicide.

Q106   The most common postpartum psychosis is of the schizophrenic type.

Q107   Severe marital problems are a poor prognostic factor in puerperal psychosis.

Q108   Postpartum depression tends to last about 1 month in 50% of cases if not treated.

Q109   Rapid cycling affective disorder affects men and women equally.

Q110   There is a blunted TSH response to TRH in depression.

Q111   Hyperparathyroidism can be a side-effect of lithium treatment.

Q112   Women who consume up to 21 units of alcohol per week are classified in the low-risk category of developing alcohol-related problems.

Q113   Approximately 10–20% of people who drink alcohol excessively develop liver cirrhosis.

Q114   Delirium tremens should be regarded as a medical emergency with a mortality rate of up to 35% if not treated.

Q115   Over 25% of inpatients on general medical wards have a psychiatric disorder.

Q116   Latah, which is found among women in Malaysia, is characterised by a period of brooding followed by violent behaviour.

Q117   Paranoid symptoms are known to occur in patients with hyperadrenalinism.

Q118   Panic attacks can be induced by an IV infusion of sodium lactate.

Q119   Global Assessment of Functioning is measured on a scale of 1–100 over a specified time period.

Q120   The use of operational definitions in DSM-IV refers to the specification of both inclusion and exclusion criteria.

Q121   It is recommended that ECT should not be used as a maintenance therapy in depression.

Q122   Blood injury phobias differ from other phobias in causing a bradycardia.

Q123   The presence of avoidance is necessary to make a diagnosis of PTSD.

Q124   Depersonalisation is a type of dissociative state.

Q125   Multiple personality disorder has been postulated to be iatrogenic.

(Q126) Insight is usually preserved in the frontal lobe syndrome.

(Q127) The single most important sign of a deep temporal lobe lesion is a contralateral lower quadrantanopia.

(Q128) Spontaneous confabulation is pathognomonic of Korsakoff's syndrome.

(Q129) Bilateral body image disturbances are commoner with left cerebral lesions than with right ones.

(Q130) Disorientation in time precedes that for place and person in dementia.

(Q131) The pathological changes in late-onset and presenile forms of Alzheimer's disease are the same.

(Q132) The degree of cognitive impairment in Alzheimer's disease correlates with synaptic loss but not with the number of neurofibrillary tangles.

(Q133) The amyloid precursor protein (APP) gene and apolipoprotein E4 are located on chromosome 21.

EMI 1

Options:

A   Denial
B   Displacement
C   Isolation
D   Projection
E   Rationalisation
F   Reaction formation
G   Splitting
H   Sublimation
I   Regression
J   Turning against self
K   Repression

From the above list, choose the **most likely** defence mechanism used in each of the following scenarios. Each scenario requires **one** answer. Each option can be used once, more than once or not at all.

Q134   A 19-year-old woman who was adopted as a child discovers the identity of her biological mother. After their first meeting, she feels anger towards her but is unable to express this directly. On returning home she cuts her wrists superficially.

Q135   A 30-year-old woman in A&E discusses her experience of being gang raped at the age of 10 years. She uses a matter-of-fact tone and shows no emotion.

Q136   During an argument, a wife is informed by her husband that he wants a divorce. When the divorce papers arrive in the post she is genuinely surprised, as she cannot recall any conversation about the impending divorce.

Q137   A 30-year-old man has recurrent thoughts about setting fire to bridges. He subsequently becomes a dedicated fire-fighter.

Q138   A shop assistant arrives home from work after one of his customers has been particularly rude to him. He then shouts furiously when his son fails to greet him.

Q139   A 20-year-old woman jumps out of a ground-floor window. When asked why she did it, she replies that the stairs were too steep and, being in a great hurry, she took the shorter route.

Q140   A woman in the outpatient clinic states 'what a caring doctor you are – the doctor I saw previously had no understanding of my problems at all'.

Q141   An aggressive young man becomes a successful heavyweight boxing champion.

Q142   During her psychotherapy session a woman describes her very disappointing experience at the benefits agency, and the therapist feels suddenly frustrated, worthless and disappointed.

EMI 2

Options:

A Anterograde amnesia for music
B Aprosody
C Colour agnosia
D Comprehension aphasia
E Dressing apraxia
F Echopraxia
G Expressive aphasia
H Finger agnosia
I Global amnesia
J Personality change
K Problem-solving difficulties
L Retrograde amnesia for music

From the above list, choose the symptom that is **most indicative** of each of the following lesions. Choose **one** answer for each. The options can be used once, more than once or not at all.

Q143 Non-dominant frontal lobe lesion.

Q144 Occipital lobe damage.

Q145 Dominant parietal lobe damage.

Q146 Non-dominant parietal lobe damage.

Q147 Left-sided temporal lobe damage.

Q148 Medial temporal lobe lesion.

Q149 Prefrontal cortex damage.

Q150 Bilateral temporal lobe damage.

EMI 3

Options:

A   Amisulpride
B   Clozapine
C   Haloperidol
D   Olanzapine
E   Quetiapine
F   Sulpiride
G   Thioridazine

Match each of the following scenarios with the **most likely** drug from the above list. The number of answers required is indicated in parentheses. Each option can be used once, more than once or not at all.

Q151   A 24-year-old man with a first episode of psychosis was commenced on this drug. A few months later he was seen in the OPC, where it was noticed he had gained a significant amount of weight. (1)

Q152   A 34-year-old woman was commenced on this drug as previous antipsychotics had failed to produce any improvement in her symptoms. However, it was soon noticed that she was constantly drooling. (1)

Q153   A 32-year-old woman was commenced on this atypical antipsychotic. A few weeks after treatment, she started complaining of breast pain and amenorrhoea. (1)

Q154   A 54-year-old patient, with a longstanding history of being treated for schizophrenia, started complaining of decreasing visual acuity, impaired night vision and brownish colouring of vision. (1)

Q155 A GP trainee in psychiatry was asked to commence antipsychotic medication in a patient with schizophrenia who had no previous history of treatment. From the list above, choose the two most unsuitable drugs for this patient. (2)

EMI 4

Options:

A CJD
B Gerstmann's syndrome
C Marchiafava–Bignami's disease
D Normal pressure hydrocephalus
E Rotor syndrome
F Shy–Drager syndrome
G Steele–Richardson–Olszewski syndrome
H Wilson's disease
I Zollinger–Ellison syndrome

Match each of the following with the **most appropriate** option from the list above. Each question requires **one** answer only. Each option can be used once, more than once or not at all.

Q156 Dyscalculia, agraphia, finger agnosia and right–left disorientation are features of this syndrome.

Q157 This is a cause of Parkinsonism and is associated with absent vertical gaze and dementia.

Q158 This condition is associated with orthostatic hypotension, Parkinsonism and an atonic bladder.

Q159 This condition is caused by widespread demyelination of the corpus callosum, optic tracts and cerebellar peduncles.

Q160 This is a disorder of copper metabolism that may result in dementia.

Q161 This condition is associated with a dementia of insidious onset with unsteady gait, psychomotor retardation and urinary incontinence.

EMI 5

Options:

A   Internal–external locus of control
B   Link between build and personality
C   Personal construct theory
D   Repertory grids
E   Self-theory
F   Stages of psychosexual development
G   Trait theory

Pair each of the following individuals with the **most appropriate** option from the list above. Each question requires **one** answer only. Each option can be used once, more than once or not at all.

Q162   Sheldon.

Q163   Bannister.

Q164   Kelly.

Q165   Freud.

Q166   Rotter.

EMI 6

Options:

A   BDI
B   Brief Psychiatric Rating Scale
C   Clinical Global Impression
D   GHQ
E   Ham-D
F   Hospital Anxiety and Depression Scale
G   Montgomery–Asberg Depression Rating Scale
H   PANSS
I   PSE
J   SCID
K   YBOCS

For each of the following indications, choose the **most appropriate** rating scale(s) from the options above. The number of answers required is indicated in parentheses. Each option can be used once, more than once or not at all.

Q167   Two instruments used to make diagnoses in research settings. (2)

Q168   The two most appropriate instruments for use in monitoring symptoms of psychosis. (2)

Q169   An instrument to screen for non-psychotic illness in primary care. (1)

Q170   An instrument to monitor obsessional and compulsive symptoms. (1)

Q171   The instrument best used for assessing psychiatric symptoms in a medical outpatient clinic. (1)

Q172   Two observer-rated depression rating scales. (2)

EMI 7

Options:

A   Anterior parietal lobe lesion
B   Dominant parietal lobe lesion
C   Dominant temporal lobe lesion
D   Frontal lobe lesion
E   Gerstmann's syndrome
F   Lesion in deep midline structures
G   Non-dominant parietal lobe lesion
H   Non-dominant temporal lobe lesion
I   Occipital lobe lesion
J   Posterior parietal lobe lesion
K   None of the above

For each of the following symptoms choose the **most likely** underlying pathology from the list above. Each question requires **one** answer only. Each option may be used once, more than once or not at all.

(Q173)   Inability to point to left ear with right index finger.

(Q174)   Difficulty in putting on trousers.

(Q175)   Finger agnosia, right–left disorientation, dyscalculia and dysphasia.

(Q176)   Contralateral lower quadrantanopia.

(Q177)   Inability to discriminate two stimuli (two-point discrimination).

EMI 8

Options:

A   Autochthonous delusion
B   Capgras syndrome
C   Cotard's syndrome
D   De Clerambault's syndrome
E   Déjà vu
F   Delusional memory
G   Delusional perception
H   Ekbom's syndrome
I   Fregoli's syndrome
J   Jamais vu
K   Morbid jealousy
L   Nymphomania

For each of the following scenarios, choose the **most appropriate** option from the list above. Each question requires **one** answer. Each option may be used once, more than once or not at all.

 A 32-year-old man gets caught up in heavy rain and suddenly realises that it was an attempt by the IRA to flood the city in order to drown him.

 A 32-year-old British news reporter on her first war project in Iraq feels as if she has been in a war situation in the past, although she acknowledges that this is not the case.

 A 32-year-old man with a 3-year history of schizophrenia claims that his recent-onset headache has resulted from the 'Z rays' he was subjected to in childhood.

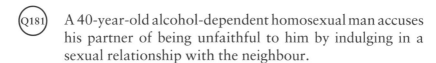 A 40-year-old alcohol-dependent homosexual man accuses his partner of being unfaithful to him by indulging in a sexual relationship with the neighbour.

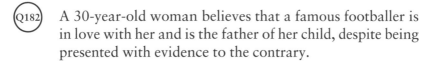 A 30-year-old woman believes that a famous footballer is in love with her and is the father of her child, despite being presented with evidence to the contrary.

Q183 A 48-year-old woman believes that her husband has been replaced by an imposter who is pretending to be her husband.

EMI 9

Options:

A   Alpha$_1$ agonism
B   Alpha$_1$ blockade
C   D$_1$ and D$_5$ receptors
D   D$_2$ and D$_3$ receptors
E   GABA$_A$ receptor
F   GABA$_B$ receptor
G   NMDA-type glutamate receptor
H   Non-NMDA-type glutamate receptor
I   5HT$_{1A}$ partial agonism
J   5HT$_{1A}$ partial blockade
K   5HT$_{2A}$ agonism
L   5HT$_{2A}$ blockade
M   5HT$_{2C}$ blockade

For each of the following drugs, choose from the list above the receptor at which it exerts its **main mechanism** of action. Each question requires **one** answer. Each option may be used once, more than once or not at all.

Q184 Baclofen.

Q185 Buspirone.

Q186 Sulpiride.

Q187 LSD.

Q188 Phencyclidine.

Q189 Diazepam.

EMI 10

Options:

A   Anankastic PD
B   Anxious (avoidant) PD
C   Dependent PD
D   Dissocial PD
E   Emotionally unstable PD (borderline type)
F   Emotionally unstable PD (impulsive type)
G   Histrionic PD
H   Paranoid PD
I   Schizoid PD

Match each of the following descriptions with the **most appropriate** diagnosis from the list above. Each question requires **one** answer. Each option may be used once, more than once or not at all.

Q190   Feelings of excessive doubt and caution.

Q191   A shallow and labile affect, with over-concern about physical attractiveness.

Q192   Outbursts of violence are common in response to criticism.

Q193   Internal preferences are often disturbed, with chronic feelings of emptiness.

Q194   Persistently bearing grudges and with an excessive sensitivity to setbacks.

Q195   Finds new activities pleasurable but has limited capacity to express feelings.

Q196   An incapacity to maintain close relationships and to feel guilt.

Paper 2:
Answers

(A1) **True.** (1: p.118)

(A2) **False.** It decreases cognitive dissonance. Cognitive dissonance is increased by low pressure to comply, greater choice of options, awareness of responsibility for actions and the expectation of unpleasant consequences. (1: p.93)

(A3) **False.** The opposite is true. (1: p.345)

(A4) **True.** Pluralistic ignorance is the misconception shared by bystanders that the situation is 'safe', due to everyone trying to conceal signs of anxiety. It is a form of inhibition produced by the presence of others. (1: p.435)

(A5) **False.** Berkowitz's research shows that it increases violence. (1: p.516)

(A6) **True.** This is Lorenz's theory, according to which aggression (like the other three instincts – hunger, sexuality and flight) does not occur in response to environmental stimuli, but builds up spontaneously and needs regular release. (1: p.516)

(A7) **False.** It measures attitudes. It contains a range of statements that are to be agreed/disagreed with. (5: p.49)

(A8) **False.** This is true in democratic leaderships. It is submissive and attention seeking in autocratic leaderships. (1: pp.290–1)

(A9) **False.** It is mental age/chronological age multiplied by 100. (1: p.589)

(A10) **True.** The other five verbal subtests are arithmetic, digit span, vocabulary, information and comprehension. (4: p.110)

(A11) **True.** Individuals read words that are spelled irregularly. Word-reading ability proves to be resistant to influences that impair other aspects of cognitive function. (4: p.111)

(A12) **True.** Idiographic theories describe personality as being individualistic and idiosyncratic. Psychoanalytic, humanistic (including personal construct theory) and cognitive–behavioural theories are of this type. (2: p.88) (19: p.566)

(A13) **True.** In hemisomatognosia, individuals do not recognise the presence of a body part, usually a contralateral limb. It occurs in temporal and parietal lobe damage. Other symptoms of non-dominant temporal lobe damage are prosopagnosia, visuospatial difficulties, impairment of learning and retention of non-verbal material (e.g. music and faces). Bilateral medial temporal lobe lesions can produce the amnestic syndrome. (4: p.18)

(A14) **False.** It was suggested by Kretschmer. Furthermore, it is schizotypal personality disorder that is believed to be related to schizophrenia. In ICD-10 it has been included in the schizophrenia chapter and is now called schizotypal disorder. (10: p.167)

(A15) **True.** Imprinting is the emotional attachment that occurs within a few minutes after birth, and it can even be to an inanimate object. It occurs in animals other than primates. (3: p.47)

(A16) **False.** It was described by Piaget. Other features of this stage include animism (believing that inanimate objects are alive), egocentrism (believing that everything happens in relation to oneself) and authoritarian morality (believing that wrong-doing should be punished according to degree of damage caused rather than intention). (3: p.51) (5: p.71)

(A17) **True.** It is also usually slower to develop in twins, large families, social classes IV and V, in cases where there is a lack of stimulation (e.g. due to deafness or neglect) or a history of IUGR, or following a prolonged second stage of labour. (3: p.52)

(A18) **False.** It is up to 20%. (7: p.67)

(A19) **True.** Also when in a multicultural society, in the absence of negative stereotypes and when the culture in the family and that in the society are congruent. (7: p.77)

(A20) **True.** As are eating disorders, alcohol and drug abuse, molestation of children and weakening of sexual identity. (3: p.49)

(A21) **False.** Although this is true of authority orientation (stage 4), the reward orientation (stage 2) is part of the pre-conventional level of morality. In the former, laws and social rules are obeyed to avoid censure of authorities and guilt about 'not doing one's duty'. In the latter, rules are conformed to in order to obtain rewards or have favours returned. (3: p.53) (6: p.85)

(A22) **False.** There are two types of associative learning, namely classical and operant conditioning. Cognitive and observational learning are distinct from this. (5: p.1)

(A23) **True.** Secondary reinforcers have achieved this status by being associated with primary reinforcers (those that satisfy basic needs, e.g. food satisfies hunger). Money can buy food, as can tokens, for example. (5: p.6)

(A24) **False.** They both develop at 4 months. (5: p.13)

(A25) **True.** This determines whether two novel objects appear the same to an infant, taking advantage of the fact that they habituate (i.e. stop looking at new objects). Both objects are presented sequentially. If the second object is perceived to be similar to the first one, the infant will have already habituated and so will spend less time looking at it. (6: pp.183–4)

A26 **False.** LTM helps to recode information so that one item covers more than one piece of information (chunking). For example, the seven digits of a telephone number can be recoded into one telephone number. Although there is a limit to the number of chunks in working memory (7 ± 2), their content is unlimited. (5: p.21)

A27 **True.** The mechanism for this is unclear, but it may be partly due to the hippocampus being immature until the age of 2 years, resulting in insufficient consolidation. (6: pp.290–1)

A28 **True.** Episodic refers to personal memories, whereas semantic refers to memory for knowledge *that* (e.g. I know *that* Big Ben is in London). (6: p.291)

A29 **True.** Extrinsic needs are those that require satisfaction externally (e.g. hunger, which requires food), whereas other needs are intrinsically satisfying (e.g. beauty). Maslow described seven levels of needs. In ascending order they are as follows: physical (e.g. hunger), safety, love and belonging, self-esteem, cognitive (to know and understand), aesthetic and the highest level of needs, namely self-actualisation. (5: p.41)

A30 **True.** As are condensation and symbolisation. (5: p.162)

A31 **False.** The structural model consists of the id, ego and superego, and it replaced his topographical model (consisting of the unconscious, preconscious and conscious). (16: p.44)

A32 **False.** It occurs between 1 and 3 years. The oral stage is from birth to 1 year, followed by the anal stage, the phallic stage (from 3 to 5 years), latency (from 6 years to puberty) and the genital stage (from puberty to early adulthood). (16: p.37)

(A33) **False.** It should be thinking rather than believing. Intuition is unconscious perception, sensation is obtaining factual information, and thinking refers to logic and reasoning. (5: pp.165–6)

(A34) **True.** And bad objects are split/projected. (16: p.103)

(A35) **False.** It is usually practised in groups. It was developed by Fritz Perls. (16: pp.179–80)

(A36) **False.** These concepts include traps, snags and dilemmas. Traps refer to the way in which individuals reinforce negative beliefs by acting in ways that elicit them. Snags lead to the inappropriate abandonment of personal aims because of a perceived negative outcome (whether true or false). Dilemmas are said to occur when there is a false dichotomisation of choices. (16: p.171)

(A37) **False.** It is structured, focused and brief. (16: p.164)

(A38) **False.** They slow down absorption. (2: p.609)

(A39) **True.** (2: p.609)

(A40) **True.** This refers to the metabolism undergone by orally ingested drugs during passage from the hepatic portal system through the liver before entering the systemic circulation. (2: p.609)

(A41) **True.** As do moclobemide, phenothiazines, SSRIs, sodium valproate, cimetidine and propranolol. (2: p.609)

(A42) **True.** As it is a cytochrome P450 inducer. (8: p.152) (9)

(A43) **False.** It is extensively metabolised in the liver but does not induce P450. (10: p.698)

(A44) **True.** On rare occasions. (9)

(A45) **False.** Sedating TCAs and related compounds include amitriptyline, clomipramine, dothiepin, doxepin, maprotiline, mianserin, trazodone and trimipramine. Those with less sedative properties include amoxapine, imipramine, lofepramine, nortriptyline and viloxazine. Protriptyline has a stimulant action. (9)

(A46) **True.** (9)

(A47) **True.** Other side-effects include drowsiness, confusion, ataxia, amnesia, dependence and paradoxical agitation. (9)

(A48) **False.** It is less sedating. Serious arrhythmias have been reported. (9)

(A49) **False.** It is only occasionally associated with them. Other side-effects include weight gain and hyperprolactinaemia (although clinical manifestations are rare in the latter). (9)

(A50) **False.** It causes both. (9)

(A51) **True.** (9)

(A52) **False.** Both can cause this. (9)

(A53) **False.** A reduced plasma thyroid concentration has been reported with quetiapine. (9)

(A54) **False.** Prolongation has been reported. (10: p.665)

(A55) **True.** It is broken down into glutamate and succinic semialdehyde, which is subsequently metabolised to succinate. (3: p.160) (11: p.312)

(A56) **True.** Other glutamate receptors include AMPA (quisqualate), kainate and the metabotropic glutamate receptor. The first two are ionotropic (ion channel linked) and the last one is G-protein and second messenger linked. (11: p.387)

(A57) **False.** Moclobemide is a reversible inhibitor of MAO_A, which metabolises 5HT and norepinephrine. MAO_B degrades phenylethylamine and benzylamine, and its inhibition is used to prevent progression in Parkinson's disease. Both types of MAO metabolise tyramine and dopamine. (3: pp.157, 178) (10: p.686) (11: p.215)

(A58) **True.** In addition to nasal congestion, sedation and a reflex tachycardia. (10: p.669)

(A59) **False.** It inhibits them at the presynaptic terminal. It inhibits reuptake of (in decreasing order of potency) 5HT, norepinephrine and dopamine. Therefore its action on 5HT is present at low doses, whilst dopamine reuptake inhibition occurs only at high doses. Inhibition of norepinephrine reuptake is thought to be associated with its anxiolytic effect. (11: pp.246–7)

(A60) **True.** It is converted to 5-hydroxytryptophan and then to 5HT (5-hydroxytryptamine) by tryptophan hydroxylase and 5-hydroxytryptophan decarboxylase, respectively. 5HT is then metabolised to 5HIAA (5-hydroxyindoleacetic acid) by MAO_A. (3: pp.158–9) (11: p.213)

(A61) **True.** Norepinephrine is metabolised to MHPG (3-methoxy-4-hydroxyphenylglycol) and VMA (vanillyl mandelic acid) by MAO and COMT (catechol-O-methyl transferase). (5: p.231)

(A62) **True.** As it is a partial agonist, any use of additional opiates results in less stimulation and muted withdrawal. (9) (11: p.522)

(A63) **True.** And also muscarinic receptors. An increase in $5HT_2$, D_1 and A_1 (adenosine purinoceptors) receptors has also been found. (3: p.186)

(A64) **True.** It refers to any change in an individual's behaviour that results from being studied. (12: pp.39, 40, 47)

(A65) **True.** Addition is the term used when the combined effect is greater than the individual effects. (12: pp.39, 40, 47)

(A66) **True.** Age disorientation is defined as a 5-year discrepancy between the patient's actual age and what the patient claims to be their age. It occurs in chronic schizophrenia. (13: p.81)

(A67) **False.** This is fantasy thinking and it occurs in normal people. (13: p.151)

(A68) **False.** It is a type of formal thought disorder described by Cameron. (13: p.160)

(A69) **True.** (13: p.168)

(A70) **True.** In depersonalisation disorder it may last a few hours, in TLE a few minutes and in anxiety disorders a few seconds. (13: p.235)

(A71) **False.** Speech is reduced in volume and associated with a cough of gradual onset (bovine cough), but without complete loss of function. It occurs in vocal cord paralysis or paresis. Inability to vocalise is called aphonia. (13: p.174) (15: p.16)

(A72) **True.** As well as infantile autism, learning disability, latah and dementia. (13: p.175)

(A73) **True.** Speech is spontaneous and fluent, and comprehension, repetition and writing are unaffected. It is also known as subcortical visual aphasia. (13: p.176)

(A74) **True.** There is a feeling that time is standing still. The same experience may occur in mania and in normal people having an exceptional experience. (13: p.83)

(A75) **False.** The stages of bereavement in chronological order are protest (stunned), preoccupation (yearning for the deceased), disorganisation (denial) and resolution (coming to terms with the loss). (3: p.58)

(A76) **False.** It has been established in both. In ICD-10, the criteria for panic disorder are several severe attacks of autonomic anxiety within a period of about 1 month, and in circumstances where there is no objective danger. These attacks are not confined to known situations, and there must be comparative freedom from symptoms between attacks. (13: p.332)

(A77) **True.** This is one of the characteristics of an obsessional symptom. (13: p.336)

(A78) **True.** They may also occur in organic psychosyndromes. (13: p.339)

(A79) **False.** They are unreasonable and inappropriate. The anxiety is associated with specific situations or objects, resulting in avoidance. (13: p.334)

(A80) **False.** They are usually not aggressive. Impulsive and aggressive acts occur in emotionally unstable and antisocial personality disorder. (13: p.353) (14)

(A81) **False.** Although violent behaviour may be seen in borderline personality disorder, it is most consistently associated with schizophrenia. (13: p.354)

(A82) **False.** They frequently have overvalued ideas. (13: p.382)

(A83) **False.** Individuals behave normally for most of the time. (13: p.385)

(A84) **True.** Furthermore, anankasts are extremely sensitive to criticism and characteristically have rigid patterns of behaviour. Anankastic personality traits are frequently observed in professionals such as doctors and lawyers. (13: p.387)

(A85) **False.** These are characteristic of anxious (avoidant) PD. Dependent PD is characterised by feelings of inadequacy, dependence upon others and a severe lack of self-confidence. (13: p.388)

(A86) **True.** These are delusions that form out of the blue and are a type of primary delusion. (13: p.123)

(A87) **False.** First-rank symptoms are thought insertion/withdrawal/broadcasting, passivity phenomena, somatic passivity, delusional perception and auditory hallucinations (third person, running commentary and thought echo). (13: p.164)

(A88) **True.** It is experienced as sinister, and the patient often feels perplexed and apprehensive, as if awaiting an impending revelation. When the delusion does finally fully form, it is usually a relief. (13: p.104)

(A89) **False.** Ekbom's syndrome describes the abnormal experience of infestation with small but microscopic organisms. It can take the form of a tactile hallucinatory state, delusion or overvalued idea, and can occur in a variety of conditions, most commonly affective psychoses. (13: p.139)

(A90) **True.** This is when images are seen from shapes (e.g. an animal in the clouds). It is involuntary, occurs more commonly in children and may also occur in pathological states (e.g. with psychotropic drugs). (13: p.97)

(A91) **True.** (13: p.88)

(A92) **True.** (13: p.96)

(A93) **True.** (13: p.107)

(A94) **False.** These are hypnagogic hallucinations. Hypnopompic hallucinations are those that occur while waking. They can be in the visual, auditory or tactile modalities. (13: p.112)

(A95) **True.** Synaesthesia occurs when a stimulus in one modality causes a perception in another (e.g. when hearing chalk scratch on a blackboard sends a shiver down your spine). Reflex hallucinations occur when a stimulus in one sensory modality causes a hallucination in another (e.g. seeing a ball bounce against a wall and feeling it against your leg). (13: p.113)

(A96) **True.** (13: p.130)

(A97) **True.** (13: p.58)

(A98) **True.** In contrast, déjà vu occurs when an event never before experienced feels strongly familiar. It can be a normal phenomenon, but it may also occur in the context of temporal lobe epilepsy and neuroses. (13: p.67)

(A99) **True.** Confabulation is the falsification of memory occurring in clear consciousness. (13: p.68)

(A100) **True.** Others include multiple personality disorder, epidemic/communicated/mass hysteria and war neurosis (shell shock). (13: pp.241–68)

(A101) **True.** (13: pp.241–68)

(A102) **False.** The reverse is true. Gender identity is the private perspective of one's own gender that is established early in life and retained by the subject, whereas gender role is the type of behaviour that an individual engages in, that identifies them as being male or female. (13: p.273)

(A103) **True.** Other disorders included are fetishism, fetishistic transvestism, exhibitionism, voyeurism and sadomasochism. (13: p.277) (14)

(A104) **True.** Sexual pleasure and gratification are derived from exposing the genitals to the opposite sex. (13: p.279)

(A105) **True.** Other risk factors are male gender, older age, living alone, social isolation, a history of previous suicide attempts and hopelessness. (17: p.151)

(A106) **False.** Around 75% of postpartum psychoses are affective. Insomnia and hyperactivity are often early symptoms, and perplexity and confusion frequently occur. (10: p.500) (17: p.379)

(A107) **True.** Others include a family history of psychiatric problems, schizophrenia and neurotic personality. (17: p.380)

(A108) **False.** The correct figure is 90%. In around 4% of cases post natal depression can last as long as 1 year if not treated. It is associated with older age, childhood separation from one's father, marital conflicts, physical problems in pregnancy and mixed feelings about the baby. (17: p.381)

(A109) **False.** There is a female preponderance. It is commonly concomitant with hypothyroidism and is usually lithium resistant. (10: p.282)

(A110) **True.** (17: p.51)

(A111) **True.** Although it is rare. Hypothyroidism is more common. (10: p.698)

(A112) **False.** Men who drink 0–21 units/week and women who drink 0–14 units/week are considered to be at low risk of developing health problems. These figures are arbitrary, however. (10: p.539)

(A113) **True.** Although rates of mortality from liver cirrhosis have decreased in some developed countries recently. There is a correlation between the rate of liver cirrhosis and mean alcohol consumption. (10: p.542)

(A114) **True.** If treated, it has a mortality rate of up to 5%. Features include clouding of consciousness, disorientation, vivid hallucinations, sweating, fever, tachycardia, raised blood pressure, mydriasis, dehydration and electrolyte disturbance. (10: p.546)

(A115) **True.** The nature and frequency of the psychiatric disorder depend upon the age and sex of the individual, in addition to the speciality of the ward. (10: p.459)

(A116) **False.** Although latah is found among women in Malaysia, it is characterised by echolalia, echopraxia and other abnormal, excessively compliant behaviour. The condition usually begins after a frightening episode. (10: p.267)

(A117) **True.** In addition, mood disorders (especially depression) commonly occur. (10: p.489)

(A118) **True.** (10: p.239)

(A119) **True.** It forms Axis V. (18: p.30)

(A120) **True.** (10: p.93)

(A121) **True.** (24: p.21)

(A122) **True.** And sometimes even fainting. This can be understood as a physiological response by the body in an effort to conserve blood pressure and minimise any potential 'blood loss'. In contrast, other phobias lead to a tachycardia (fight or flight response). (14)

(A123) **False.** The required criteria are onset within 6 months of a traumatic event with repeated reliving of this in flashbacks, intrusive memories, daytime imagery or dreams. Emotional detachment, numbing of feeling and avoidance of stimuli reminiscent of the trauma are often present, but not essential for the diagnosis. (14)

(A124) **False.** It is not classified as such because only limited aspects of personal identity are usually affected. (14)

(A125) **True.** In this rare disorder, two or more distinct personalities exist within an individual, with only one being evident at a time. In the most common form of two personalities, one is usually dominant and both are almost always unaware of each other's existence. (14)

(A126) **False.** Insight, especially concern for the future and consequences of actions, is limited, leading to gross errors of judgement. (20: p.964)

(A127) **False.** Upper quadrantanopias result from temporal lobe lesions, whereas lower quadrantanopias result from parietal lobe lesions. (20: p.966)

(A128) **False.** Korsakoff described two types of confabulation. The spontaneous or fantastic type is seen in the early stages of Wernicke–Korsakoff syndrome and frontal lobe pathology. Momentary or provoked confabulation consists of fleeting intrusion errors or distortions in response to a memory test, and can be found in approximately 50% of Korsakoff patients. Neither is pathognomonic of Korsakoff's syndrome. (20: p.968)

(A129) **True.** (20: p.975)

(A130) **True.** (10: p.406)

(A131) **True.** (10: p.623)

(A132) **False.** It correlates with both. (10: p.623)

(A133) **False.** APP is on chromosome 21 and apolipoprotein E4 is on chromosome 19. (10: p.623)

EMI 1

Reference for all (16: pp.21–8)

(A134) **J.** This is when an impulse that is meant to be expressed is turned against the self.

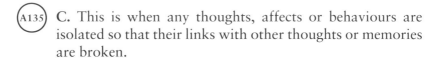

(A135) C. This is when any thoughts, affects or behaviours are isolated so that their links with other thoughts or memories are broken.

(A136) A. This is denying external reality, usually when it is painful or unwanted.

(A137) F. This is to take up an attitude that is completely opposite to the original one.

(A138) B. This is when ideas, emotions or thinking are transferred from their original object to a more acceptable substitute.

(A139) E. This is when attempts are made to explain ideas or thoughts in a logical way. It occurs in normal people and in delusional symptoms.

(A140) G. This is the complete division of 'good' qualities, affects and memories from 'bad' ones (segregating things into 'black' and 'white').

(A141) H. This is to channel the forces of unacceptable instincts (e.g. aggression) into creative or acceptable activities.

(A142) D. This is when difficult or unwanted thoughts or feelings are projected on to another person.

EMI 2

(A143) B. Prosody is the emotional aspect of speech. (3: p.31)

(A144) C. (4: p.18)

(A145) H. (4: p.18)

(A146) E. (4: p.18)

(A147) D. (4: p.18)

(A148) **A.** (4: p.18)

(A149) **K.** Other abilities affected are perceptual judgement, memory and planning. Personality change occurs in cases of orbital cortex damage. (5: p.61)

(A150) **I.** (4: p.18)

EMI 3

(A151) **D.** (9)

(A152) **B.** (9)

(A153) **A.** This woman had hyperprolactinaemia. This is particularly reported with amisulpride, and is characterised by galactorrhoea, gynaecomastia and sexual dysfunction. (9)

(A154) **G.** Thioridazine (a group 2 phenothiazine) may rarely cause pigmentary retinopathy (at high doses) in addition to prolongation of the QT interval. If there is prolonged use of the drug, monitoring for visual defects is advised, as are ECG and electrolyte measurement (before commencing treatment and at 6-month intervals). (9)

(A155) **B, G.** Neither is recommended as first-line treatment for schizophrenia or other psychotic states. Clozapine is licensed for schizophrenia in patients who are unresponsive to or intolerant of conventional antipsychotics. Thioridazine may only be prescribed under specialist supervision as a second-line treatment for schizophrenia. (9)

EMI 4

(A156) **B.** It is caused by dominant parietal lobe lesions. (5: p.61)

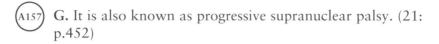

(A157) **G.** It is also known as progressive supranuclear palsy. (21: p.452)

(A158) **F.** It is also known as multi-system atrophy. (21: p.452)

(A159) **C.** This syndrome is a consequence of alcoholism, and is associated with ataxia, epilepsy, dysarthria and marked impairment of consciousness. (10: p.544)

(A160) **H.** It is also known as hepatolenticular degeneration, and is due to an autosomal recessive gene on chromosome 13. This causes copper deposition in the liver and brain, among other organs. (21: p.712)

(A161) **D.** CT scan of the head reveals dilated ventricles without cortical atrophy; CSF pressure is normal. It is caused by an obstruction to outflow from the subarachnoid space. (5: p.551)

EMI 5

(A162) **B.** He described the endomorphic (viscerotonic), ecto-morphic (cerebrotonic) and mesomorphic (somatotonic) personality types. (5: p.468)

(A163) **D.** These can be used to assess attitudes and formal thought disorder by means of a series of bipolar constructs. (5: p.39)

(A164) **C.** Kelly believed that individuals interpret the world on the basis of past experience. (5: p.31)

(A165) **F.** (5: p.164)

(A166) **A.** Rotter postulated that individuals vary along a dimension of locus of control. Internal locus is associated with more confidence about changing one's life and the environment. (5: p.468)

EMI 6

 I, J. The SCID (Structured Clinical Interview for DSM-IV) is a semi-structured interview that looks at past and present illness. The PSE (Present State Examination) is a structured mental state interview that measures symptoms in the previous month. (19: p.156)

 B, H. The Brief Psychiatric Rating Scale is widely used in the management of psychotic symptoms and psychopathology, as it can be completed quickly. The Positive and Negative Symptoms Scale is more detailed and structured, and so takes longer to complete. (19: p.159)

 D. The General Health Questionnaire is a 60-item, self-administered tool that takes approximately 15 minutes to complete (shorter versions are also available). It refers to symptoms within the last 4 weeks. Scoring above the cut-off indicates that psychiatric morbidity is likely, but does not equate with a diagnosis. (19: p.155)

 K. The Yale–Brown Obsessive-Compulsive Scale is observer rated. (10: p.68)

 F. This is a 14-item scale. (19: p.162)

 E, G. The Hamilton Depression Scale is a widely employed observer-rated tool used in research. It measures severity of depression rather than being a diagnostic instrument. The Montgomery–Asberg Depression Rating Scale is a 10-item observer-rated scale that only scores psychological symptoms. (10: pp.67–8) (19: pp.159–61)

EMI 7

Reference for all (20: pp.964–9)

 B. Finger agnosia and right–left disorientation.

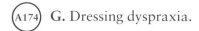

(A174) **G.** Dressing dyspraxia.

(A175) **K.** This is not Gerstmann's syndrome as, although there is finger agnosia, right–left disorientation and dyscalculia, dysgraphia is not present. Gerstmann's syndrome results from a dominant parietal lobe lesion.

(A176) **J.**

(A177) **A.**

EMI 8

(A178) **G.** In this case, the subject experienced a normal perception (rain), which he then interpreted with a delusional meaning (IRA involvement) that had immense personal significance (to drown him). Unlike autochthonous delusions (delusional intuition), which occur in a single stage, delusional perception occurs in two stages, namely perception followed by false interpretation. (13: p.123)

(A179) **E.** Unfamiliar experiences seem familiar in déjà vu, whereas the opposite occurs in jamais vu. (13: p.234)

(A180) **F.** In delusional memory the subject recalls as 'remembered' an event or idea (e.g. receiving 'Z rays') that is clearly delusional in nature. (13: p.126)

(A181) **K.** Jealousy is particularly prominent in homosexual couples, since the insecurity of a liaison that is not sanctioned by convention or law is especially likely to result in suspicion. (13: pp.132–3)

(A182) **D.** Delusions of love include erotomania and De Clerambault's syndrome. They are different from uncontrolled sexual desire in women (nymphomania) and men (satyriasis). (13: p.133)

A183 **B.** Other delusional misidentification syndromes include intermetamorphosis, subjective doubles and Fregoli's syndrome. (13: p.134)

EMI 9

A184 **F.** It is an agonist, used for the relief of chronic muscle spasm and spasticity. (12: p.76)

A185 **I.** Unlike a full agonist, it does not produce the maximum effect. (12: p.74)

A186 **D.** This is a benzamide and it is selective for D_2 and D_3 receptors. (12: p.308)

A187 **K.** The hallucinogenic effects of LSD are decreased by $5HT_{2A}$ antagonists (some atypical antipsychotics). (12: p.74)

A188 **G.** Like amphetamine, phencyclidine and ketamine produce hallucinations and delusions, but in addition may cause negative-like symptoms, such as blunted affect and emotional withdrawal. (10: pp.356–7)

A189 **B.** (12: p.285)

EMI 10

A190 **A.** Other features include preoccupation with rules and lists; task completion is often interfered with due to the need to achieve perfection. (14)

A191 **G.** Other features include self-dramatisation, suggestibility and inappropriate seductiveness. (14)

A192 **F.** Other features include emotional instability and lack of control. (14)

A193 **E.** There are also intense unstable relationships, excessive efforts to prevent abandonment and threats of suicide or deliberate self-harm. (14)

A194 **H.** Other features include suspiciousness (specifically regarding the fidelity of partners), misconstruing actions as hostile and having a tenacious sense of personal rights. (14)

A195 **I.** There is also emotional coldness, detachment, indifference to praise or criticism, a lack of desire for close friends and insensitivity to social norms. (14)

A196 **D.** There is also persistent irresponsibility, a low tolerance of frustration and a low threshold for aggression/violence. (14)

Paper 3:

Questions

(Q1) According to cognitive dissonance theory, dissonance will occur only when volitional behaviour is involved.

(Q2) Polytropic attachment is more common than monotropic attachment.

(Q3) In terms of conditioning, discrimination is brought about by differential reinforcement.

(Q4) Stereotyping is the process of ascribing characteristics to individuals on the basis of their group membership.

(Q5) Piaget described the sensorimotor stage of cognitive development as being when the child develops causal relationships with the outside world.

(Q6) According to social exchange theory, our attitudes towards other people are determined by our estimate of the rewards they can offer.

(Q7) Working memory includes the phonological buffer and visual–spatial sketchpad.

(Q8) Diffusion of responsibility is a factor that will determine help by a bystander in an emergency situation.

(Q9) In language development, a child would normally be expected to speak 8–10 words by the age of 12 months.

(Q10) Semantic differential scales have poor test–retest reliability.

(Q11) Exchange relationships tend to be more insecure and cause more dissatisfaction than communal relationships.

(Q12) Approximately 25% of children have an eidetic memory.

(Q13) Personal construct theory is an example of an idiographic theory of personality.

(Q14) The General Health Questionnaire is suitable for detecting psychoses.

(Q15) Implicit messages are more persuasive in less intelligent recipients.

(Q16) The average age of onset of puberty in males is 2.5 years later than that in females.

(Q17) The Thematic Apperception Test is self-rated.

(Q18) Stimulation of the medial hypothalamus results in hunger.

(Q19) Visual and tactile sensory memory are known as iconic and haptic memory, respectively.

(Q20) Triangulation within the family can cause discord.

(Q21) The concrete operational stage usually develops in adolescence.

(Q22) Ideomotor apraxia is a symptom of parietal lobe damage.

(Q23) Forgetting from LTM is usually a result of decay rather than failure of retrieval.

(Q24) The Hamilton Rating Scale for Depression assesses symptoms in the last 7 days.

(Q25) Dressing apraxia is a symptom of dominant parietal lobe damage.

Q26 Object permanence refers to knowing the existence of objects that are out of sight.

Q27 The Wisconsin Card Sorting Test is a test of executive function.

Q28 The Hamilton Anxiety Scale is self-rated.

Q29 Crystallised intelligence continues to grow throughout adult life.

Q30 According to social learning theory, aggression is learned by modelling.

Q31 Weber's law states that the increase in stimulus strength required to enable two stimuli to be perceived as different is directly proportional to the value of the initial strength of the stimulus.

Q32 Systematic desensitisation is a two-stage process.

Q33 The preconscious uses primary process thinking whereas the conscious operates via secondary process thinking.

Q34 The ego, which is mostly conscious, is at the centre of object relations.

Q35 The superego develops in response to parental rewards and punishments.

Q36 Transference refers to the therapist's own feelings and emotions.

Q37 The conscience and the ego-ideal are components of the superego.

Q38 Jung founded the school of analytic psychology.

(Q39) The objective psyche, also known as the collective unconscious, was defined by Berne.

(Q40) Castration anxiety is a phenomenon that appears in both Freudian and Kleinian theory.

(Q41) Ataxia is a known side-effect of lithium at therapeutic doses.

(Q42) Partial agonists, such as buspirone, do not induce the maximal response at their receptor sites.

(Q43) Lithium may cause vomiting, but not diarrhoea.

(Q44) St John's wort increases the anticoagulant effect of warfarin.

(Q45) Carbamazepine given with lithium causes neurotoxicity at therapeutic doses.

(Q46) Weight gain is a known side-effect of phenelzine.

(Q47) The $GABA_B$ receptor is a chloride channel that has recognition sites for both benzodiazepines and barbiturates.

(Q48) Barbiturates are hepatic enzyme inducers.

(Q49) Nortriptyline is an inactive metabolite of amitriptyline.

(Q50) Isocarboxazid is an MAOI.

(Q51) A regular dose of any drug takes twice its half-life to achieve steady-state plasma concentration.

(Q52) Acutely ill patients show lower response rates to placebo treatment than those who are chronically ill.

(Q53) Psychosis, hallucinations and aggressive behaviour have all been reported with the use of sertraline.

Q54 First-order elimination kinetics are said to occur when the rate of drug elimination is proportional to its concentration.

Q55 The cheese reaction is due to tyramine-stimulated release of norepinephrine.

Q56 LSD is a $5HT_{2A}$ partial agonist.

Q57 SSRIs inhibit the cytochrome P450 enzyme.

Q58 Acetylcholine esterase synthesises acetylcholine from acetyl CoA and choline.

Q59 Chlordiazepoxide has a more sustained duration of action than lorazepam.

Q60 Lofexidine, an $alpha_1$-receptor antagonist, is used in the symptomatic treatment of heroin withdrawal.

Q61 Risperidone is a potent antagonist at both D_2 and $5HT_2$ receptors.

Q62 Naltrexone is an opiate agonist used in the treatment of heroin withdrawal.

Q63 Carbamazepine induces its own metabolism.

Q64 Panic and phobia occur more frequently together than separately.

Q65 Intermetamorphosis is a type of delusional misidentification syndrome, in which it is believed that a familiar person is taking on different appearances.

Q66 Personal construct theory has been used to investigate disorder of thought.

Q67 Circumstantial thinking is a form of thought disorder.

Q68 Panic disorder is also known as 'episodic paroxysmal anxiety'.

Q69 Illness phobia is the same as hypochondriasis.

Q70 Almost all factitious disorders can be included in the term malingering.

Q71 Body image distortion in anorexic patients is a perceptual abnormality.

Q72 Subjects with transvestism wear clothes of the opposite sex for the purpose of sexual excitement.

Q73 Dysmorphophobia most commonly takes the form of an overvalued idea.

Q74 In hebephrenic schizophrenia attention is not affected.

Q75 The word 'paranoid' in psychiatric terminology means self-referent.

Q76 Free-floating anxiety is a term used to describe anxiety that is attached to floating objects.

Q77 In affective illness, abnormalities of volition are associated with abnormalities of activity.

Q78 Depersonalisation is an unpleasant experience with an affective component.

Q79 Elementary hallucinations typically occur in organic states.

Q80 Mania à potu may occur after drinking only a small amount of beer.

Q81 Distortion of the experience of time occurs in depersonalisation.

Q82   Impulsive and aggressive acts are uncommon in schizophrenia.

Q83   The twilight state is usually an organic condition that lasts for a few hours to several weeks.

Q84   Paraphasia is a pattern of speech in which the last syllable of a word is repeated.

Q85   Periodic somnolescence with overeating occurs in the Kleine–Levin syndrome.

Q86   'I can feel oil inside my brain' would be an example of a hygric hallucination.

Q87   Pseudologia fantastica occurs in antisocial personality disorder.

Q88   Gilles de la Tourette's syndrome is more common in boys, usually starting between the ages of 10 and 12 years.

Q89   Echolalia is a symptom of latah.

Q90   The embarrassment (momentary) type of confabulation is more common than the fantastic variety.

Q91   Negative autoscopy occurs when an individual cannot see their image in a mirror.

Q92   Obstruction is the equivalent of thought block occurring in the flow of action.

Q93   Dissocial PD should not be diagnosed unless the subject is over 16 years of age.

Q94   In conduction dysphasia, spontaneous speech is affected.

Q95   Delusional atmosphere is a type of primary delusion.

(Q96) Individuals with histrionic PD have great difficulty in sustaining a long-term, mutually rewarding relationship.

(Q97) Vorbeigehen, or approximate answers, is a feature of Ganser's syndrome.

(Q98) Delusional patients tend to make excessive external, stable and global attributions of negative events.

(Q99) Men are more sensitive than women to the harmful effects of alcohol.

(Q100) Around 60% of individuals suffering from schizophrenia commit suicide within 6 months of discharge from hospital.

(Q101) Schizotypal personality disorder features in both ICD-10 and DSM-IV.

(Q102) The highest consumption of alcohol is generally among young married men.

(Q103) Above the age of 50 years, more women than men present with DSH.

(Q104) Prominent defence mechanisms and learning disability can be categorised on Axis II of DSM-IV.

(Q105) Following an act of DSH, 10% of cases will commit suicide within the next year.

(Q106) The earliest and commonest feature of alcohol withdrawal is sweating.

(Q107) ICD-10 is available in a simpler format for primary healthcare.

(Q108) Psychosocial and environmental problems over the last 2 years can be recorded on Axis IV of DSM-IV.

Q109 The prodrome of puerperal psychosis usually begins hours after parturition.

Q110 A significant proportion of people who are dependent on alcohol are also dependent on benzodiazepines.

Q111 In depression, there is failure of dexamethasone suppression.

Q112 Unilateral ECT is associated with a greater incidence of side-effects than is bilateral ECT.

Q113 Factitious disorders account for 15% of referrals to psychiatric liaison services.

Q114 Over-generalisation is a defence mechanism.

Q115 Lupus, Addison's disease and thyroid disorders are recognised organic causes of depression.

Q116 In PTSD, exposure to aversive memories is central to treatment.

Q117 Mild mania is frequently reported in patients on steroid therapy.

Q118 Dissociative amnesia, unlike dissociative fugue, is sudden in onset and slow in termination.

Q119 Tongue-biting occurs in 50% of patients with pseudoseizures.

Q120 With regard to obsessional rituals, slowness without repetition is more common in women.

Q121 Night terrors occur in REM sleep.

Q122 Witzelsucht is inappropriate jocularity associated with the frontal lobe syndrome.

Q123 Eye movement desensitisation has been advocated as a treatment for hypochondriacal disorder.

Q124 Denial of blindness is a characteristic feature of Anton's syndrome.

Q125 Dysphasia is uncommon in parietal lobe lesions.

Q126 Unilateral body image disturbances are more common with right than with left hemisphere lesions.

Q127 Fluctuating impairment of consciousness is a feature of dementia with Lewy bodies.

Q128 Depression is invariable in the later stages of dementia.

Q129 Schizoaffective disorder is more common in women.

Q130 Women with premenstrual syndrome are more likely to suffer from comorbid depression and anxiety.

Q131 A history of psychiatric problems is a risk factor for abnormal grief reaction.

Q132 In women, bipolar II disorder is more common than bipolar I disorder.

Q133 La belle indifference may be seen in psychogenic aphonia.

EMI 1

Options:

A   Chunking
B   Decay
C   Eidetic memory
D   Episodic memory
E   Explicit memory
F   Implicit memory
G   Priming
H   Proactive interference
I   Retrieval failure
J   Retroactive interference
K   Semantic memory
L   Storage failure

For each of the following scenarios, choose the **most appropriate** option from the list above. The number of answers required is indicated in parentheses. Each option can be used once, more than once or not at all.

Q134   Remembering the events of your first day at medical school. (1)

Q135   Remembering the way home from work. (1)

Q136   Knowing that Big Ben is in London and remembering that you visited it last night. (2)

Q137   The 'tip-of-the-tongue' experience. (1)

Q138   Finding it difficult to remember the position of your newly changed permanent parking space within the same car park. (1)

Q139   Remembering the digits 7984621 as the phone number of your grandmother. (1)

Q140   Forgetting the date of a meeting you have just set, because you became distracted by a discussion with a colleague. (1)

Q141   Remembering how to tie your shoelaces. (1)

EMI 2

Options:

A   Agranulocytosis
B   Cardiac arrhythmia
C   Dry mouth
D   Hyperprolactinaemia
E   Hypersalivation
F   Nausea
G   Postural hypotension
H   Urinary retention
I   Vomiting
J   Weight gain

Match each of the following with the **most appropriate** side-effect from the list above. Each question requires **one** answer. Each option may be used once, more than once or not at all.

Q142   This anti-adrenergic side-effect is especially important in the elderly.

Q143   This well-recognised side-effect of olanzapine can precipitate an endocrine disorder.

Q144   This is a well-known side-effect of antipsychotics, but clinical manifestations of this condition are rare with olanzapine.

Q145   This is a potentially fatal condition and is particularly associated with clozapine.

Q146   This anticholinergic side-effect can cause severe abdominal discomfort and even presentation to the A&E department as an emergency.

Q147   This side-effect, which is particularly associated with clozapine and zotepine, can be treated with hyoscine.

EMI 3

Options:

A Amphetamine
B Cannabis
C Heroin
D Phencyclidine
E 3 units of alcohol
F 4 units of alcohol
G 5 units of alcohol
H 6 units of alcohol
I 12 units of alcohol

Match each of the following with the **most appropriate** option from the list above. Each question requires **one** answer. Each option may be used once, more than once or not at all.

 Q148 This compound has both stimulant and mild hallucinogenic properties.

 Q149 The number of units in 3 pints of ordinary-strength beer.

 Q150 The number of units in 3 measures of vodka.

EMI 4

Options:

A Delirium tremens
B Dementia in Alzheimer's disease
C Dementia in CJD
D Dementia in HIV
E Dementia in Huntington's disease
F Dementia in Parkinson's disease
G Dementia in Pick's disease
H Lewy body dementia
I Multi-infarct dementia
J Normal pressure hydrocephalus

For each of the following scenarios, choose the **most likely** option from the list above. Each question requires **one** answer. Each option may be used once, more than once or not at all.

 A 72-year-old man is referred to your clinic. The GP letter states that his family have recently noticed a decline in his memory. On examination he has a pill-rolling tremor and cogwheel rigidity, which he has had for several years.

 A 65-year-old man with a history of recent onset of forgetfulness, falling over and urinary incontinence is referred to your clinic. The CT scan reveals dilated ventricles with no cortical atrophy.

 A 55-year-old man has been referred to your clinic because he has been masturbating in public. He also has rapid mood swings and is generally irritable. The CT scan reveals fronto-temporal atrophy.

 A 71-year-old man presents to the A&E department with visual hallucinations, delusions and cognitive impairment.

He also has features that suggest an acute confusional state. He developed severe EPSEs when he was given 0.5 mg of risperidone.

EMI 5

Options:

A   Arterial hypertension
B   Chronic physical illness
C   Ethnic minority background
D   Female gender
E   Feelings of hopelessness
F   Impaired vision
G   Lack of a confidant
H   Loss of mother before the age of 11 years
I   Premorbid schizoid personality
J   Recent discharge from a psychiatric inpatient unit
K   Feelings of worthlessness

For each of the following conditions, choose the **most appropriate** risk factors from the list above. The number of answers required is indicated in parentheses. Each option can be used once, more than once or not at all.

 Suicide. (3)

 Depression. (4)

 Late-onset schizophrenia. (3)

EMI 6

Options:

A   Acanthocytosis
B   High serum copper level
C   Hypercalcaemia
D   Hyperglycaemia
E   Hyponatraemia
F   Hypophosphataemia
G   Increased mean corpuscular volume
H   Increased 24-hour urinary catecholamines level
I   Low serum caeruloplasmin level
J   Low serum copper level
K   Low serum vitamin B$_6$ level
L   No response to Synacthen
M   Macrocytosis

Match each of the following scenarios with the **two most appropriate** options from the list above. Each option may be used once, more than once or not at all.

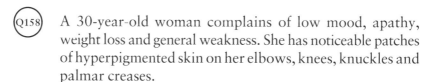 A 30-year-old woman complains of low mood, apathy, weight loss and general weakness. She has noticeable patches of hyperpigmented skin on her elbows, knees, knuckles and palmar creases.

Q159   A 17-year-old man presents with a coarse tremor, dysphagia and muscular rigidity. On physical examination, jaundice and hepatomegaly are found. The family complains that his personality has changed.

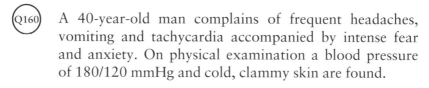 A 40-year-old man complains of frequent headaches, vomiting and tachycardia accompanied by intense fear and anxiety. On physical examination a blood pressure of 180/120 mmHg and cold, clammy skin are found.

A 60-year-old man complains of low mood, anhedonia, fatigue, severe constipation and anorexia. He also reports increased thirst, polyuria, muscle weakness, dull headaches and lumbar back pain.

EMI 7

Options:

A   Anhedonia
B   Apolipoprotein E4
C   Cold intolerance
D   Disinhibition
E   Euphoria
F   Features of UMN lesion
G   Mental retardation
H   Negative automatic thoughts
I   Presenelin 1 and 2
J   Repeated falls
K   Transient ischaemic attack
L   Visual hallucinations

For each of the following scenarios, choose the **two most likely** options from the list above. Each option can be used once, more than once or not at all.

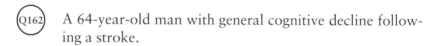 A 64-year-old man with general cognitive decline following a stroke.

A 74-year-old woman with fluctuating consciousness and marked sensitivity to neuroleptics.

A 70-year-old woman with gradual cognitive decline and impairment of language and memory.

A 60-year-old man with persistent low mood, forgetfulness and poor attention.

A 70-year-old man with prominent behavioural and emotional disturbances, but with relatively preserved memory and general intellect.

EMI 8

Options:

A   Amitriptyline
B   Citalopram
C   Dothiepin
D   Fluoxetine 20 mg/day
E   Fluoxetine 60 mg/day
F   Fluvoxamine
G   Imipramine
H   Moclobemide
I   Nortriptyline
J   Paroxetine
K   Sertraline
L   Tranylcypromine
M   Venlafaxine
N   Venlafaxine XL

For each of the descriptions below, choose the treatment(s) **licensed in the UK** from the above list of options. The number of answers required is indicated in parentheses. Each option may be used once, more than once or not at all.

 A 7-year-old child with a history of involuntary voiding of urine at night for several months. After thorough investigation, no underlying organic cause is found. (3)

 A 19-year-old woman with a BMI of 19 presents with a history of self-induced vomiting. On questioning, she admits to overeating and being excessively preoccupied with the control of her body weight. (1)

 A 33-year-old woman experiencing symptoms of anxiety and depression only during the late luteal phase of her menstrual cycle. (1)

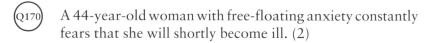 A 44-year-old woman with free-floating anxiety constantly fears that she will shortly become ill. (2)

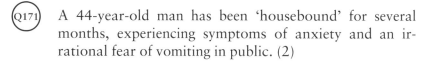 A 44-year-old man has been 'housebound' for several months, experiencing symptoms of anxiety and an irrational fear of vomiting in public. (2)

EMI 9

Options:

A Depersonalisation
B Derealisation
C Dissociative disorder
D Factitious disorder
E Generalised anxiety disorder
F Hypochondriasis
G Social phobia
H Somatisation disorder

For each of the following scenarios, choose the **most appropriate** diagnosis. Choose **one** answer for each scenario. Each option can be used once, more than once or not at all.

 A young woman complains about being under a lot of stress. She reports frequently feeling detached, as if she was 'watching herself from the outside emotionlessly'.

 A 40-year-old man complains of abdominal pain for the last 7 months and is convinced that he has pancreatic cancer. Extensive gastroenterological investigations do not show any abnormalities. He will not accept reassurance from physicians.

 A 32-year-old woman complains of non-specific aches and pains, palpitations, sweating and flushing which started 3 years ago following separation from her husband. She asks for medication to relieve her symptoms. She has had various specialist investigations for a variety of different symptoms, but no organic cause has been found.

A young woman drives away after collecting the result of her failed examination. She buys petrol and eats in various restaurants without any overt problems. She returns home after several days but has no recollection of her journey.

EMI 10

Options:

A Adjustment disorder
B Amok
C Epilepsy
D Evil eye
E Frigophobia
F Koro
G Latah
H Panic attack
I Schizophrenia
J Voodoo
K Windigo

For each of the following scenarios choose **one** of the above options. Each option may be used once, more than once or not at all. Note that for all of the following patients, physical examination and relevant investigations revealed no abnormalities.

 A week after his mother's death, a Pakistani man suddenly started complaining that his penis was retracting into his abdomen, which he thought would result in his death.

 A young Asian man was seen running down the street, rubbing his face, screaming and throwing objects at passers-by. This resulted in admission to a psychiatric ward. Two days after recovery, he reported witnessing someone setting fire to his warehouse prior to admission.

 An Asian woman was brought to A&E, where it was reported that she had been following her relatives around at home while imitating their speech and movements. Of note was the huge financial loss she had incurred a fortnight ago.

A middle-aged man reported being frightened of turning into a man-eater after hearing about his family's death in a road traffic accident.

Paper 3:
Answers

(A1) **True.** When we believe we have no choice, there is neither dissonance nor attitude change. (1: p.355)

(A2) **False.** Monotropic attachment occurs when attachment is to one individual. It is more common than polytropic attachment. (5: p.25)

(A3) **True.** Discrimination is recognising that two similar stimuli are in fact different. (6: pp.237–8)

(A4) **True.** (1: p.332)

(A5) **True.** The sensorimotor stage occurs from birth to 2 years of age. At the age of 4 months the child develops discretionary smiling, at 8 months they develop purposeful behaviour, and at 12 months they develop object permanence. There are three subsequent stages, namely pre-operational (2–7 years), concrete operational (7–12 to 14 years) and formal operational (12–14 years onwards). (3: p.51)

(A6) **True.** (1: p.411)

(A7) **True.** The phonological buffer briefly stores information in an acoustic code, whereas the visual–spatial sketchpad does so in a visual or spatial code. (6: p.275)

(A8) **True.** The greater the number of people present, the less likely a bystander is to help. (1: pp.435–7)

(A9) **False.** Spoken language develops as follows: 3 months, babbling; 9 months, repetitive babbling; 12 months, 3 words; 18 months, 20–40 words. (3: p.52)

(A10) **False.** They have good reliability. (1: p.352)

(A11) **True.** According to social exchange theory, in communal relationships rewards are given out of thoughtfulness for the other. Such relationships tend to be happier than the exchange type, where couples keep mental records of 'gifts'. (1: p.417)

(A12) **False.** Around 5% do. This is more commonly known as a photographic memory. (5: p.17)

(A13) **True.** Idiographic theories describe personality as being individualistic and idiosyncratic. Psychoanalytic, humanistic (including personal construct theory) and cognitive–behavioural theories are of this type. (2: p.88) (19: p.566)

(A14) **False.** It is not suitable for this purpose. It is designed as a screening instrument for use in primary care or for community surveys in order to detect neurosis. It can be completed within 10 minutes and has subscales for somatic symptoms, anxiety, insomnia, depression and social functioning. (10: p.68)

(A15) **False.** They are more persuasive in more intelligent recipients. (5: p.51)

(A16) **False.** The average age of onset of puberty in females is 11 years, compared with 11.5 years for males. In girls the first sign is usually breast development, whereas in boys it is usually gonadal enlargement. (3: p.56)

(A17) **False.** It is a projective test of motivation and personality in which the individual is shown ambiguous pictures and asked to make up the story. (1: p.129)

(A18) **False.** Hunger occurs if the lateral hypothalamus is stimulated. The medial hypothalamus is a satiety centre. (5: p.40)

(A19) **True.** Sensory memory for auditory information is known as echoic memory. (5: p.17)

(A20) **True.** Triangulation refers to the presence of exclusive relationships within the family. Other causes of discord are communication problems, overprotection, rejection and enmeshment. (5: p.28)

(A21) **False.** It develops between the ages of 7 and 11 years. During this stage, children develop logical thought and are able to perform operations, such as being able to understand the laws of conservation. (3: p.51)

(A22) **True.** This is the inability to carry out progressively more difficult tasks. It occurs in both dominant and bilateral parietal lobe damage. (2: p.19) (4: pp.18, 57)

(A23) **False.** The reverse is true. (5: p.22)

(A24) **True.** It has a maximum score of 50, and a score of 30 or above indicates severe depression. It is observer rated and measures the severity of symptoms in individuals who have already been diagnosed. (10: p.67)

(A25) **False.** It is a symptom of non-dominant parietal lobe damage. Other symptoms include anosognosia, hemisomatognosia and prosopagnosia. (4: p.18)

(A26) **True.** Object permanence was described by Piaget. This gradually develops at 1 year of age during the sensorimotor stage of development. (7: p.62)

(A27) **True.** It is used to test for frontal lobe lesions. (2: p.383)

(A28) **False.** It is observer rated. It measures the severity of anxiety symptoms; some depressive symptoms are included. (10: p.67)

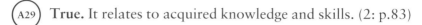

(A29) **True.** It relates to acquired knowledge and skills. (2: p.83)

(A30) **True.** (1: pp.516–18)

(A31) **True.** However, it is only an approximation and does not hold true at extremes of stimulus intensity. (5: p.10)

(A32) **True.** Initially relaxation training is taught, which is then used in the second stage of exposure. (5: p.7)

(A33) **False.** Both the preconscious and conscious operate via secondary process thinking. It is the unconscious that operates via primary process thinking. (16: p.47)

(A34) **False.** The ego is mainly unconscious. Other functions include rational thinking, reality testing, external perception, voluntary motor action and the activation of defence mechanisms. (16: p.44)

(A35) **True.** It is concerned with morality and approximates to the conscience. Although the superego is more conscious than the id, most of its functions are still unconscious. (16: p.45)

(A36) **False.** This describes counter-transference. (16: pp.58–60)

(A37) **True.** The conscience punishes the ego (e.g. with guilt), whereas the ego-ideal rewards it (e.g. with praise). (16: p.45)

(A38) **True.** (16: p.100)

(A39) **False.** Berne was involved in the development of transactional analysis. It was Jung who described this phenomenon. (16: pp.100, 107)

(A40) **True.** (2: p.559) (5: p.167)

(A41) **False.** This occurs at toxic doses. Other toxic effects include CNS disturbances such as mild drowsiness and sluggishness, coarse tremor and dysarthria. (9)

(A42) **True.** Buspirone is a partial agonist at the $5HT_{1A}$ receptor. (11: pp.85, 273)

(A43) **False.** It can cause both. (9)

(A44) **False.** It decreases it (as it is an enzyme inducer). (9)

(A45) **True.** (9)

(A46) **True.** Adverse effects commonly associated with MAOIs include postural hypotension (especially in the elderly) and dizziness. Less commonly these drugs cause weight gain. (9)

(A47) **False.** This is true of the $GABA_A$ receptor, which also has recognition sites for zopiclone and zolpidem. (11: pp.312–13)

(A48) **True.** (2: p.610)

(A49) **False.** It is an active metabolite. (2: p.610)

(A50) **True.** As are phenelzine and tranylcypromine. (9)

(A51) **False.** It takes more than five times its half-life. (9)

(A52) **False.** The reverse is true. (12: pp.39, 40, 47)

(A53) **True.** As has amnesia. (9)

(A54) **True.** (2: p.611)

(A55) **True.** It is associated with MAOI use and can result in a potentially fatal rise in blood pressure. Tyramine, which is normally broken down by MAO (A and B), enters the circulation and stimulates prolonged release of norepinephrine. This is exacerbated by decreased metabolism of the latter, again due to MAO inhibition. (11: pp.215–16)

(A56) **True.** As are the other hallucinogens psilocybin, mescaline and MDMA. (11: p.512)

(A57) **True.** Especially fluoxetine. (8: p.15)

(A58) **False.** It breaks down acetylcholine to form choline and acetic acid. It is inhibited by the antidementia drugs donepezil, galantamine and rivastigmine. It is choline acetyltransferase (CAT) that synthesises acetylcholine from acetyl CoA and choline. (3: pp.150–2)

(A59) **True.** Diazepam also has a sustained action. Lorazepam and oxazepam are shorter-acting compounds. (9)

(A60) **False.** Although it is used in this way, it is an alpha$_2$ agonist and thus acts presynaptically. Therefore, when activated, it reduces the norepinephric surge seen in heroin withdrawal. (9) (10: p.568)

(A61) **True.** As is olanzapine (although it has comparatively slightly weaker D$_2$ antagonism). In contrast, clozapine has low D$_2$/high 5HT$_2$ affinity, and quetiapine has low D$_2$/low 5HT$_2$ affinity. Risperidone also acts as an antagonist at alpha$_1$, alpha$_2$ and H$_1$ receptors. (10: p.665)

(A62) **False.** It is a non-selective opiate antagonist used to maintain abstinence after detoxification. Individuals should be opioid free for at least 7–10 days. (3: p.188) (9)

(A63) **True.** Other liver enzyme inducers include barbiturates, alcohol, phenobarbitone, phenytoin, primidone, rifampicin and cigarette smoking. (3: p.186) (11: p.211)

(A64) **True.** There is considerable overlap between the neurotic symptoms. (13: p.329)

(A65) **False.** This describes Fregoli's syndrome, one of the four types of delusional misidentification syndromes. The others include Capgras syndrome (in which it is believed that a familiar person has been replaced by a double), intermeta-morphosis (in which a familiar person and a stranger are believed to be physically and psychologically identical) and subjective doubles (in which another person is believed to have been physically but not psychologically transformed into his or her own self). (13: p.134)

(A66) **True.** It was originally described by Kelly and can be investigated experimentally using the repertory grid. (13: p.161)

(A67) **False.** It occurs characteristically in epilepsy, learning disability and obsessional personalities. (13: p.154)

(A68) **True.** (13: p.332)

(A69) **False.** Illness phobia is an unreasonable fear of developing illness, whereas hypochondriasis is a preoccupation with symptoms. (13: pp.241–68)

(A70) **False.** Malingering is driven by an external incentive such as financial compensation, whereas the subject with factitious disorder assumes a sick role in which the motivation is almost always obscure. Munchausen's syndrome is classified within the category of factitious disorders. (14)

(A71) **False.** It is usually an overvalued idea. (13: pp.241–68)

(A72) **True.** (13: p.278)

(A73) **True.** (13: p.143)

(A74) **False.** It is disturbed. (13: p.163)

(A75) **True.** The word 'paranoid' refers to all beliefs that are self-referential, not just those that are persecutory. (13: p.144)

(A76) **False.** This is when the anxiety state is not attached to any specific provoking factor. (13: p.330)

(A77) **True.** In depressive states retardation is prominent, whereas overactivity is seen in mania. (13: p.346)

(A78) **True.** There is emotional numbing. (13: p.230)

(A79) **True.** Elementary (simple) hallucinations consist of unstructured noises such as music or machinery. They are experienced as unpleasant or frightening. (13: p.100)

(A80) **True.** During this condition, senseless violence occurs, followed by a prolonged period of sleep and total or partial amnesia. It is also known as pathological intoxication. (13: p.47)

(A81) **True.** (13: p.231)

(A82) **False.** They are not uncommon in schizophrenia, although they tend to be over-represented in crime statistics for violence. (13: p.355)

(A83) **False.** In ICD-10 it is classified as a dissociative condition that starts and finishes abruptly, lasting from a few hours to several weeks. (13: p.46)

(A84) **False.** It is the production of an inappropriate sound in place of a word or phrase. Repetition of syllables is called logoclonia and it occurs in Parkinson's disease. (13: p.173)

(A85) **True.** This syndrome is characterised by intense hunger with overeating and periodic somnolence. Although the combination of sleep and appetite disturbance suggests a hypothalamic disorder, there is no conclusive evidence for this. (13: p.345)

(A86) **True.** These are superficial tactile hallucinations in which there is a perception of fluid. Other types of superficial hallucinations are haptic (perception of touch) and thermic (perception of heat and cold). (13: p.106)

(A87) **True.** It is also known as fluent plausible lying and may occur in histrionic PD as well. (13: p.173)

(A88) **False.** Although it is more common in boys, onset is usually between the ages of 5 and 8 years. A history of motor before vocal tics is characteristic. (13: p.369)

(A89) **True.** Latah is a dissociative disorder. Symptoms include hypersensitivity to sudden noise, echopraxia, echolalia, automatic responses to commands and dissociative behaviour. It affects the Malay and Iban people, predominantly women. (2: p.334)

(A90) **True.** These are the two types of confabulation. The embarrassment type occurs when a patient confabulates in an attempt to cover up a memory deficit of which they are aware. The fantastic type occurs when the patient spontaneously recounts experiences of a fantastic and unbelievable nature. Both types most commonly occur early in Korsakoff's syndrome (and subsequently disappear with declining cognitive functioning). (13: pp.67–8)

(A91) **True.** (13: p.111)

(A92) **True.** (13: p.365)

(A93) **False.** It should not be diagnosed unless the subject is over the age of 18 years. (13: p.384)

(A94) **False.** Speech remains fluent. Although comprehension is normal, repetition and naming are abnormal. (13: p.177) (15: p.17)

(A95) **True.** As are delusional perception, autochthonous delusions and delusional memory. (13: p.123)

(A96) **True.** Although acquaintanceships are easily and rapidly formed. In addition, they have inconsistent and fluctuating moods, crave attention and are inconsiderate of others. The characteristic phenomenological disturbance is a limited ability to experience profound affect and to communicate such feelings. (13: p.386)

(A97) **True.** This is when an individual deliberately chooses to pan over a correct answer and selects a false one (e.g. answering blue in response to the question 'What colour is grass?'). Other features are clouding of consciousness, conversion symptoms and sometimes pseudohallucinations. It is a dissociative disorder. (13: p.74)

(A98) **True.** And excessively internal, stable and global attributions for positive events. (13: p.130)

(A99) **False.** Women are more sensitive to these effects due to their lower lean body mass, resulting in higher blood alcohol levels per unit consumed. (5: p.336)

(A100) **True.** Risk factors include being young, being male, having multiple relapses, high educational achievement, good premorbid functioning and depression at the last contact with services. (17: p.150)

(A101) **False.** It only features in DSM-IV (as does narcissistic PD). (18: p.641)

(A102) **False.** Although alcohol consumption by women has greatly increased over the last 15 years, it remains highest among young men who are unmarried, separated or divorced. (10: p.541)

(A103) **False.** The ratio is 1:1. (17: p.154)

(A104) **True.** As can personality disorders/personality patterns. Axis I is for clinical disorders, Axis III is for general medical conditions, Axis IV is for psychosocial and environmental conditions and Axis V is for global assessment of functioning. (18)

(A105) **False.** Approximately 1% will do so. (17: p.155)

(A106) **False.** It is tremor. Nausea, sweating and retching are frequent, and insomnia is also common. Individuals may be agitated and easily startled. (10: p.543)

(A107) **True.** It is also available in different versions for clinical work and research. (10: p.99)

(A108) **False.** Over the last year only. (18: p.29)

(A109) **False.** It usually begins after 2 days. (17: p.380)

(A110) **True.** Benzodiazepine use is extremely widespread. Most long-term users are older women; in younger people it is often used intravenously along with other illicit substances. (10: p.571)

(A111) **True.** As demonstrated by the dexamethasone suppression test. Failure of dexamethasone suppression also occurs in a variety of other conditions, such as schizophrenia, alcoholism and anorexia nervosa. (17: p.51)

(A112) **False.** The opposite is true. The commonest side-effects include memory disturbance, post-treatment confusion and headache. (19: p.896)

(A113) **False.** Although the prevalence of factitious disorders is not clear, they account for about 1% of referrals to these services. Presentations are diverse, with both physical and psychological symptoms. (10: p.473)

(A114) **False.** It is one of Beck's cognitive distortions and occurs in depression. Other distortions are minimisation, magnification, personalisation, arbitrary inference and selective abstraction. (2: p.307)

(A115) **True.** Any chronic illness can be associated with depression. (10: p.478)

(A116) **True.** This is irrespective of the type of therapy used. (5: p.417)

(A117) **True.** Paranoid symptoms are less common. Lithium prophylaxis may be considered in those who need to continue on steroid therapy. (10: p.489)

(A118) **False.** Dissociative states are reported to be sudden in both onset and termination. (14)

(A119) **False.** It is rare, as is urinary incontinence and serious bruising from falling. Loss of consciousness is absent or replaced by a state of stupor or trance. (14)

(A120) **False.** It is more common in men. Hand-washing rituals are more common in women. (14)

(A121) **False.** They occur in stages 3 to 4 of non-REM sleep. (17: p.209)

(A122) **True.** It refers to inappropriate jokes, puns or pranks. (20: p.964)

(A123) **False.** It has been advocated as a treatment for PTSD. Inducing involuntary multisaccadic eye movements while an individual is experiencing intrusive thoughts has been postulated to stop symptoms of PTSD. (10: p.198)

(A124) **True.** In Anton's syndrome there is cortical blindness with denial of disability. The individual behaves as if they can see and, when tested, describes purely imaginary experiences. It is a type of anosognosia. (4: pp.69, 379)

(A125) **False.** Dominant parietal lobe lesions produce dysphasia. (20: p.968)

(A126) **True.** (20: p.975)

(A127) **True.** And it must be differentiated from delirium. (10: p.405)

(A128) **False.** Retained insight in the early stages may result in distress and reactive depression, but emotional responses become blunted in the later stages. (10: p.406)

(A129) **True.** (17: p.375)

(A130) **True.** The premenstrual syndrome starts a few days before and ends shortly after a menstrual period. It is characterised by anxiety, irritability, food cravings and low mood. The physical symptoms include breast tenderness and a feeling of abdominal discomfort and distension. (2: p.338)

(A131) **True.** As are an inability to express grief, low self-esteem, loss of a child, loss of parents in childhood, sudden unexpected death, multiple deaths, an ambivalent or dependent relationship with the deceased, insecure attachment with the deceased, social isolation and an absent or unsupportive family. (2: p.296)

(A132) **True.** (2: p.297)

(A133) **True.** This is calm acceptance of serious disability, which may be striking, but is not universal. It is seen in dissociative disorders of movement and sensation, and also in normal individuals facing serious physical illness. (14)

EMI 1

(A134) **D.** Episodic memory refers to memory for personal episodes (autobiographical memory). (6: p.292)

(A135) **F.** Implicit (non-declarative) memory refers to knowledge of *how* to do things. It consists of memory for skills, in addition to being involved in priming, conditioning and non-associative learning (such as habituation and sensitisation). It occurs without conscious recollection of the experiences that led to the improvement. (6: pp.289–91)

(A136) **D, K.** Semantic memory refers to memory for facts, i.e. knowing *that*. . . (e.g. knowing *that* Big Ben is in London). The latter half of the question is an example of episodic memory. (6: p.292)

(A137) **I.** This can be conceptualised as failure of retrieval from long-term memory. (6: p.282)

(A138) **H.** Old learning (i.e. knowing the location of your previous permanent parking space) interferes with new learning (i.e. remembering the location of your new parking space). (6: p.283)

(A139) **A.** Seven pieces of information (each digit) are recorded using long-term memory into one chunk (the telephone number). (6: p.276)

(A140) **C.** Information from working memory is lost by decay within 20 seconds unless rehearsed. (5: p.22)

(A141) **F.** (6: p.289)

EMI 2

(A142) **G.** As it may lead to falls. (9)

(A143) **J.** A high BMI has been associated with various physical complications, including diabetes. Mild and transient anticholinergic side-effects have also been associated with olanzapine. (9)

(A144) **D.** Hyperprolactinaemia is particularly reported with amisulpride. (9)

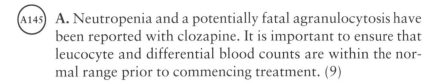

(A145) **A.** Neutropenia and a potentially fatal agranulocytosis have been reported with clozapine. It is important to ensure that leucocyte and differential blood counts are within the normal range prior to commencing treatment. (9)

(A146) **H.** Other anticholinergic effects include dry mouth, blurred vision, constipation and reduced sweating. Glaucoma may rarely be precipitated. (10: p.669)

(A147) **E.** Other side-effects of clozapine include anticholinergic and anti-adrenergic side-effects, a potentially fatal agranulocytosis, ECG changes, diabetes and myocarditis. (9) (15: p.148)

EMI 3

(A148) **D.** Phencyclidine is chemically related to ketamine (which has both anaesthetic and analgesic effects). (5: p.262) (10: p.575)

(A149) **H.** 1 pint of ordinary-strength beer contains 2 units of alcohol. (10: p.540)

(A150) **E.** 1 measure of spirits contains 1 unit of alcohol. (10: p.540)

EMI 4

(A151) **F.** This diagnosis should be considered in patients with extrapyramidal signs of Parkinson's disease who later develop dementia, especially of the subcortical type. (5: p.550)

(A152) **J.** There is normal CSF pressure; it is caused by obstruction to outflow from the subarachnoid space. (5: p.551)

(A153) **G.** Half of all cases show a family history. The mean duration of disease is 11 years. (5: p.540)

(A154) H. (5: p.550)

EMI 5

(A155) **B, J, K.** (5: p.400)

(A156) **B, D, G, H.** (5: pp.392–3)

(A157) **D, F, I.** Impaired hearing or vision contributes to social isolation and subsequent suspiciousness. There is usually no abnormality of affect, thought disorder or catatonic symptoms. (5: p.559)

EMI 6

(A158) **E, L.** Addison's disease. (4: p.518) (23: p.726)

(A159) **I, J.** Wilson's disease. (23: p.872)

(A160) **D, H.** Phaeochromocytoma. Plasma and urinary levels of vanillyl mandelic acid (VMA), metadrenaline and metnoradrenaline are elevated. (4: p.520)

(A161) **C, F.** Primary hyperparathyroidism. (4: p.528) (23: p.718)

EMI 7

Reference for all (10: pp.420, 622, 625)

(A162) **F, K.** Vascular dementia.

(A163) **J, L.** Dementia with Lewy bodies.

(A164) **B, I.** Dementia in Alzheimer's disease.

(A165) **A, H.** Depressive episode.

D, E. Dementia in Pick's disease (a fronto-temporal dementia).

EMI 8

References for all (8: pp.110–17) (14) (19)

 A, G, I. Nocturnal enuresis.

 E. Bulimia nervosa.

 D. Premenstrual tension syndrome (ICD-10). Premenstrual dysphoric disorder (DSM-IV).

 J, M. Generalised anxiety disorder.

 H, J. Social phobia.

EMI 9

 A. (13: p.230)

 F. In hypochondriasis, the individual either believes that they have an underlying serious illness or is preoccupied with a presumed deformity or disfigurement. Reassurance is not accepted, and there are repeated requests for investigations. (14)

 H. In somatisation disorder, the emphasis is on the symptoms themselves rather than on having an underlying disease. The individual asks for treatment to remove the symptoms. (14)

 C. Dissociative fugue. (14)

EMI 10

Reference for all (13: p.268)

(A176) F.

(A177) B.

(A178) G.

(A179) K.

Other culture-bound syndromes

Frigophobia: This is an obsessive-compulsive neurosis seen in East Asia. Features include a morbid fear of the cold, preoccupation with loss of vitality and the compulsive wearing of layers of clothes.

Evil eye: This is a phobic neurosis seen in Mexico (where it is believed that strong glances are harmful) and North Africa (where precautions are taken to avoid or counteract the evil eye).

Voodoo: This is the belief that violation of a taboo may result in death. It is a phobic neurosis seen in Haiti.

Paper 4:
Questions

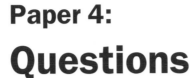

Q1 If a stimulus is redundant, in that it is already providing information that an organism knows, it will not be conditioned to the unconditioned stimulus.

Q2 Monotropic attachment is accomplished by 3 months of age.

Q3 Feedback from facial expression does not increase the intensity of emotion.

Q4 Forgetting from LTM is usually as a result of decay rather than failure of retrieval.

Q5 Separation between 6 months and 3 years of age has little effect on attachment behaviour.

Q6 In sensory perception, top-down processing becomes particularly important with unambiguous stimuli.

Q7 Circular reactions were described by Piaget as being repeated involuntary motor activities.

Q8 Two-sided messages are more likely to produce attitude change in less educated audiences.

Q9 At 6–8 months of age, fear of heights is a normal phenomenon.

Q10 The Cannon–Bard theory states that perceived emotional stimuli undergo hypothalamic processing.

Q11 At 4 years of age, a child with normal language development would be expected to use grammar correctly.

Q12 Intelligence tests are affected by situational factors such as hostility towards the assessor.

Q13 Priming is when prior exposure to a stimulus facilitates its processing on repeat exposure.

Q14 Both negative and positive life events are stressful.

Q15 Operant conditioning, also known as instrumental learning, is learned by trial and error.

Q16 Prejudice can be reduced by having personal contact with the subject of prejudice.

Q17 Memories associated with strong emotions are more easily remembered than emotionally neutral memories, because of increased rehearsal and organisation.

Q18 The Holmes and Rahe Social Readjustment Scale ranks death of a spouse as the most stressful life event.

Q19 Thurstone's primary mental abilities include numerical fluency.

Q20 Bonding and attachment are usually from infant to mother.

Q21 The Montgomery–Asberg Depression Rating Scale includes questions on somatic symptoms.

Q22 Interpersonal attraction is enhanced by proximity.

Q23 Predictability and controllability are two situational factors that can help to reduce stress.

Q24 The Ames room exemplifies the concept of size constancy.

Q25   The Brief Psychiatric Rating Scale is suitable for rating mild neurotic disorders.

Q26   Anosognosia is a symptom of dominant parietal lobe damage.

Q27   Single-parent families are associated with a higher incidence of child abuse.

Q28   Altruism is a form of helping in which the motive is to benefit the recipient.

Q29   Negative reinforcement decreases the occurrence of a behaviour by using an aversive stimulus.

Q30   According to gestalt psychology, the law of dissimilarity refers to dissimilar items being grouped apart.

Q31   Maternal deprivation between 6 months and 3 years of age is associated with enuresis.

Q32   Groupthink occurs when there is a submissive leader.

Q33   It is true to say that as some facial expressions are universally recognised, they can be said to be innate.

Q34   According to Beck's theory of depression, arbitrary interference is one of the cognitive distortions.

Q35   Klein considered the analysis of child's play to be equivalent to free association.

Q36   The 'good enough mother' is a concept associated with Winnicott.

Q37   The symbiotic phase is the first stage in Margaret Mahler's theory of development.

Q38 Being actively suicidal is a relative contraindication to explorative psychotherapy.

Q39 Primal therapy is associated with Wilhelm Reich.

Q40 Foulkes is associated with analysis 'in the group'.

Q41 Grief and role transition are two foci of interpersonal therapy.

Q42 According to Adler, 'masculine protest' in women is a reaction to their inferior position in society.

Q43 Milan developed systemic family therapy.

Q44 Dopamine, in contrast to 5HT, is a catecholamine.

Q45 Barbiturates can cause paradoxical excitement.

Q46 MAOIs can cause central nervous system toxicity if given with methadone.

Q47 Abnormal LFTs have been reported with the use of paroxetine, but not fluoxetine.

Q48 Diazepam may cause an increase in aggression.

Q49 Sulpiride is not associated with jaundice or skin reactions, unlike chlorpromazine.

Q50 Mianserin exerts its main antidepressant effect by inhibiting norepinephrine reuptake.

Q51 Lithium carbonate in therapeutic doses causes increased beta waves on EEG.

Q52 Desipramine is a metabolite of amitriptyline.

Q53 Chlorpromazine increases the plasma level of TCAs.

(Q54) Moclobemide does not cause galactorrhoea.

(Q55) Diazepam potentiates the effects of GABA by binding to the $GABA_A$ receptor.

(Q56) Epinephrine receptors are ion channels.

(Q57) Disulfiram inhibits acetaldehyde hydroxylase, resulting in symptoms of flushing, headache and nausea when taken with alcohol.

(Q58) Gabapentin, like lithium, is excreted unchanged via the kidneys.

(Q59) Maprotiline has less anticholinergic effects than imipramine.

(Q60) Lithium-induced oedema may respond to dose reduction.

(Q61) Both the urinary retention and postural hypotension caused by amitriptyline are mediated via peripheral acetylcholine receptors.

(Q62) GABA is synthesised from glutamate by glutamic acid hydroxylase.

(Q63) Serum creatinine concentration is a better measure of renal function than creatinine clearance.

(Q64) Clozapine has a higher affinity for D_4 than for D_2 or D_3 receptors.

(Q65) Clozapine serum level is reduced by caffeine.

(Q66) The difference in improvement seen in depressed patients on active treatment compared with those on placebo is greatest in the first 2 weeks.

(Q67) A pint of ordinary-strength beer contains 2 units of alcohol.

Q68   In the UK, alcohol misuse-related problems account for 10% of all psychiatric admissions.

Q69   MDMA has stimulant as well as hallucinogenic properties.

Q70   Confusion is a clinical feature of puerperal psychosis.

Q71   Concrete thinking is a pathognomonic feature of schizophrenia.

Q72   There is always a change in mood when experiencing depersonalisation.

Q73   Asyndesis is a form of thought disorder.

Q74   Approximate answers are a feature of dissociative disorders.

Q75   In pure word deafness, an individual's speech is affected.

Q76   Validity is increased by specifying characteristic rather than discriminating symptoms.

Q77   Muscle pain and poor concentration are typically present in individuals with chronic fatigue syndrome.

Q78   Kinaesthetic hallucinations are types of tactile hallucinations.

Q79   Panoramic recall may be a feature of temporal lobe epilepsy.

Q80   Phaeochromocytoma and hypoglycaemia are causes of anxiety.

Q81   Chronic feelings of emptiness, intense and unstable relationships and efforts to avoid abandonment are features of emotionally unstable personality disorder (borderline type).

(Q82) Formication is particularly associated with cocaine withdrawal.

(Q83) The clinical features of obsessional personality disorder are explained psychodynamically by the defence mechanisms of rejection, regression and reaction formation.

(Q84) In nominal aphasia, comprehension and repetition are abnormal.

(Q85) Pseudohallucinations are under voluntary control.

(Q86) Obsession is both an individual symptom and an important feature of OCD.

(Q87) The content of delusions is dictated by the type of illness.

(Q88) Phobias, like obsessions, are resisted unsuccessfully and regarded by the subject as senseless and irrational.

(Q89) Autoscopic hallucinations usually last for several hours.

(Q90) Overvalued ideas may be obsessional.

(Q91) In dysmegalopsia, objects appear larger than their real size.

(Q92) Oneirophrenia is a type of delusional disorder.

(Q93) Delusional perception, a first-rank symptom, is a two-step process.

(Q94) In depression, will is impaired more than motivation.

(Q95) Hearing a voice saying 'get lost' when a door slams is an example of a functional hallucination.

(Q96) Somatisation disorder is synonymous with the Masquerade syndrome.

Q97 In dysmorphophobia, the subject's dissatisfaction with their appearance is usually based upon the opinion of others.

Q98 There is no clouding of consciousness in epileptic automatisms.

Q99 There is no difference in meaning between the words 'gender' and 'sex'.

Q100 Distractibility refers to the simultaneous occurrence of inattention and poor concentration.

Q101 Narcolepsy is associated with hypnagogic hallucinations, sleep paralysis and catalepsy.

Q102 Pseudologia fantastica is usually associated with paranoid and antisocial personality disorder.

Q103 Dermatozoenwahn is also known as alcoholic hallucinosis.

Q104 Paramnesia is inaccuracy of memory recall.

Q105 In OCD, autonomic anxiety is often present.

Q106 Bestiality and exhibitionism are often seen in violent men.

Q107 Catatonic schizophrenia was originally described by Kahlbaum.

Q108 Learning theory would suppose that aggression is an acquired reaction that occurs in response to internal stimuli.

Q109 Tics are rapid, repetitive, uncoordinated and stereotyped movements.

Q110 Blumer and Benson described 'pseudodepressed' and 'pseudopsychopathic' types of frontal lobe syndromes.

Q111 Personality is not affected in parieto-temporal lobe lesions.

Q112 Primary or working memory is severely impaired in the amnesic syndrome.

Q113 Subjects with transsexualism experience genital excitement as a result of wearing clothing of the opposite sex.

Q114 Astereognosis and agraphaesthesia are impairments of the perception of touch.

Q115 Around 90% of those who commit suicide have a history of deliberate self-harm.

Q116 Speech dominance and handedness determine on which side the electrodes are placed in unilateral ECT.

Q117 The clinical picture in dementia is partly determined by premorbid personality.

Q118 The course of generalised anxiety disorder tends to be constant.

Q119 Language and learning are relatively preserved in subcortical dementia.

Q120 It is not possible to make a diagnosis of PTSD if the onset of symptoms is longer than 6 months after the traumatic event.

Q121 Mixed personality disorders are more common than single personality disorders.

Q122 Psychogenic tunnel vision is less common than dissociative deafness.

Q123 The essential phenomenological abnormality of dissocial personality disorder is one of empathy.

(Q124) La belle indifference may be seen in psychogenic aphonia.

(Q125) Rigid patterns of behaviour are characteristic in histrionic PD.

(Q126) The multiple sleep latency test is a diagnostic tool for narcolepsy.

(Q127) REM sleep occurs after stage 4 of non-REM sleep.

(Q128) The peak age of onset of psychotic depression is 50–70 years.

(Q129) Life events contribute equally to the onset and relapse of schizophrenia.

(Q130) Sleep spindles occur in stage 1 of non-REM sleep.

(Q131) Relapse rates of depression are more frequent following discontinuation of ECT than following discontinuation of antidepressant treatment.

(Q132) Around 30% of women experience postpartum 'blues'.

(Q133) Post-schizophrenic depression is classified under mood disorders in both ICD-10 and DSM-IV.

EMI 1

Options:

A   Difficult child
B   Easy child
C   Parents who are homosexual couples
D   Parents with a permissive style of parenting
E   Parents with an authoritarian parenting style
F   Parents with an authoritative parenting style
G   Single-parent family
H   Slow to warm up child

Match each of the following with the **most appropriate** option from the list above. Each question requires **one** answer. Each option may be used once, more than once or not at all.

Q134   This is associated with a higher incidence of child abuse.

Q135   Parents who have definite rules which children are expected to follow. The children's views are valued.

Q136   Parents who are reluctant to punish inappropriate behaviour.

Q137   Parents who have strict and enforced rules where there is little room for discussion.

Q138   Families who may experience social stigma, but no adverse effect on child development has been reported.

Q139   Children who cry a lot and are socially inhibited, unpredictable and highly active.

EMI 2

Options:

A   Age 8 months to 1 year
B   Age 1 to 3 years
C   Age 3 to 5 years
D   Age 6 to 7 years
E   Age 6 to 11 years
F   Adolescence
G   Early adulthood

Match each of the following with the **most appropriate** option from the list above. Each question requires **one** answer. Each option may be used once, more than once or not at all.

Q140   Stranger anxiety usually develops in this age group.

Q141   Erikson defined industry versus inferiority in this age group.

Q142   Erikson defined initiative versus guilt in this age group.

Q143   Gender constancy is usually achieved in this age group.

Q144   Fear of failure and social gatherings may be prominent in this age group.

EMI 3

Options:

A   Alfred Adler
B   Anna Freud
C   Carl Gustav Jung
D   Carl Rogers
E   Donald Winnicott
F   Margaret Mahler
G   Melanie Klein
H   Sigmund Freud
I   Wilfred Bion

Match each of the following concepts with the appropriate name from the list of options above. Choose **one** answer for each question. Each option can be used once, more than once or not at all.

Q145   Birth order contributes to a sense of inferiority in individuals.

Q146   The recurrence of universal symbols, which are found in myths, legends and dreams, represents manifestations of the collective unconscious.

Q147   The manifest content of dreams frequently seems absurd.

Q148   A basic need for positive regard drives every individual to strive for self-actualisation.

Q149   A basic assumption, such as pairing, interferes with creative change and development in a group.

Q150   A child must pass through a symbiotic phase before becoming separated from their mother and developing a sense of being an individual.

EMI 4

Options:

A   Advertence
B   Automatic obedience
C   Echopraxia
D   Mitgehen
E   Negativism
F   Obstruction
G   Opposition
H   Psychological pillow
I   Waxy flexibility

Match each of the following descriptions with the **most appropriate** option from the list above. Each question requires **one** answer. Each option may be used once, more than once or not at all.

Q151   The patient imitates the interviewer's every action.

Q152   The patient carries out every command in a literal and concrete fashion.

Q153   The interviewer can move the patient's limbs by directing him with fingertip pressure.

Q154   While carrying out a motor act, the patient stops in his tracks.

Q155   The limbs of the patient can be put in any posture by the interviewer and they will remain in that position for a significant period of time.

Q156   The patient turns towards the examiner when addressed, but in a bizarrely exaggerated manner.

EMI 5

Options:

A 1 week
B 2 weeks
C 1 month
D 2 months
E 3 months
F 6 months
G 1 year
H 2 years
I None of the above

To make a confident ICD-10 diagnosis for each of the following disorders, choose the duration of illness required from the list of options above. Choose only **one** option. Each option may be used once, more than once or not at all.

Q157 Simple schizophrenia.

Q158 Schizotypal disorder.

Q159 Delusional disorder.

Q160 Mania without psychotic symptoms.

Q161 Obsessive-compulsive disorder.

Q162 Somatisation disorder.

EMI 6

Options:

A   Enlarged lateral ventricles
B   Insidious onset
C   Male gender
D   Negative symptoms
E   Older age at onset
F   Paranoid type of illness
G   Prominent affective illness
H   Sudden onset
I   Younger age at onset

Match each of the following with the **most appropriate** option(s) from the list above. The number of answers required is indicated in parentheses. Each option may be used once, more than once or not at all.

 Q163   Factors predicting good prognosis in schizophrenia. (4)

 Q164   Factors predicting poor prognosis in schizophrenia. (5)

 Q165   Factors predicting good prognosis in anorexia nervosa. (1)

 Q166   Factors predicting poor prognosis in depressive disorders. (1)

EMI 7

Options:

A   Anosmia
B   Ataxia
C   Babinski sign positive
D   Encephalopathy
E   Headache
F   Increased sensitivity to noise
G   Motor aphasia
H   Parkinsonian symptoms
I   Peripheral neuropathy
J   Urinary incontinence

From the above list, choose the symptoms that are **most characteristic** of each of the following conditions. **Two** answers are required for each question. Each option may be used once, more than once or not at all.

Q167   Post-concussional syndrome.

Q168   Cerebrovascular accident.

Q169   Recurrent head injury in boxers.

Q170   Meningioma of the frontal lobe.

Q171   Lead poisoning.

EMI 8

Options:

A   Citalopram
B   ECT
C   Flupenthixol depot
D   Imipramine
E   Low-dose amisulpiride
F   Low-dose lorazepam
G   Sleep hygiene

For each of the following scenarios, choose the **most appropriate** treatment from the list of options above. Choose **one** answer for each scenario. Each option can be used once, more than once or not at all.

 A 75-year-old woman with moderately severe dementia, who lives in a nursing home, refuses to go to bed at night.

 An 80-year-old man with a history of benign prostatic hypertrophy complains of a 3-month history of low mood, anhedonia, fatigue and poor appetite. He denies weight loss.

 A 75-year-old woman with a history of recurrent falls starts seeing visions of burglars in her house and hearing the voice of her husband talking to her.

 A depressed 75-year-old woman refuses to take her medication, eat or drink. She is socially withdrawn and has difficulty sleeping.

EMI 9

Options:

A   Alcohol abuse
B   Alcohol use
C   Benzodiazepine use
D   Cannabis intoxication
E   Cannabis withdrawal
F   Cocaine intoxication
G   Cocaine withdrawal
H   LSD use
I   MDMA use
J   Opiate dependence
K   Opiate withdrawal

Match each of the following scenarios with the **most appropriate** option from the list above. Choose **one** answer for each scenario. Each option may be used once, more than once or not at all.

 A 23-year-old woman with a history of illicit drug use is brought to A&E after having a seizure. On examination her pulse is 102, her BP is 180/110 and there is evidence of nasal congestion. She is expressing grandiose and persecutory delusions about being a movie star and claims she is being prevented from marrying George Clooney.

 A 19-year-old woman presents to A&E with anxiety, social withdrawal and flashbacks. She appears distracted during interview, and a cough and reddened conjunctivae are noted.

 A 48-year-old man, who presents with profuse sweating, agitation and tachycardia, reports hearing music in his head when he sees the colour red. His answers are noticeably delayed.

A 30-year-old man presents to A&E complaining of anxiety, restlessness and non-specific aches and pains. Shivering, rhinorrhoea and lacrimation are also evident.

EMI 10

Options:

A   Abrupt onset
B   Early personality change
C   Gradual onset
D   Hypertension
E   Myoclonus
F   Parkinsonian symptoms
G   Perseveration of speech
H   Sensitivity to antipsychotics
I   Step-wise progress
J   Urinary incontinence
K   Visual hallucinations

Match each of the following diagnoses with **three** of the **most appropriate** options from the list above. Each option can be used once, more than once or not at all.

 Lewy body dementia.

 Vascular dementia.

 Pick's disease.

Paper 4:

Answers

(A1) **True.** The critical factor in learning is that there is a predictive relationship. (6: pp.238–9)

(A2) **False.** It is accomplished by 6 months of age. (3: p.46)

(A3) **False.** It can do so. This is known as the facial feedback hypothesis. (6: p.408)

(A4) **False.** The reverse is true. (5: p.22)

(A5) **False.** Secure attachment behaviour develops during the first 3 years of life. This is characterised by the child being distressed upon separation from the attachment figure, seeking contact and comfort on their return, and being able to use the attachment figure as a secure base from which to explore the environment. (3: p.47)

(A6) **False.** With ambiguous stimuli (e.g. when in a dark room). Top-down processing is driven by a person's knowledge and expectations (e.g. recognising a knife because someone is cutting vegetables with it), in contrast to bottom-up processing, which is driven by the sensory input (e.g. recognising a knife because of its handle, shape or serrated edge). (6: pp.167–8)

(A7) **False.** They are voluntary motor activities (e.g. shaking a toy). These occur from around 2 months of age and are part of the sensorimotor stage of development. (5: p.32)

(A8) **False.** Better educated people are more able to facilitate conflicting information. They may also not want to think of themselves as being easily led. (5: p.51)

(A9) **True.** At 3–5 years of age, common fears are those of animals, the dark and monsters. At 6–11 years there is fear of shameful social situations such as ridicule. (5: p.35)

(A10) **False.** They undergo thalamic processing. This theory postulates that subsequently, both the physiological and emotional responses occur together. (5: p.42)

(A11) **True.** At this age, language comprehension is better than expression. By 5 years, language is like adult speech. (3: p.52)

(A12) **True.** They are also affected by arousal, anxiety, lack of motivation, physical difficulties and familiarity with the test material. (2: p.85)

(A13) **True.** (6: p.290)

(A14) **True.** Although negative life events seem to impact more on health. (6: p.496)

(A15) **True.** Several trials are required. (5: p.3)

(A16) **True.** It can also be reduced by contact with non-stereotypic individuals, achievement of equality, a collaborative effort and an environment that supports equality. (1: p.365)

(A17) **True.** (5: p.22)

(A18) **True.** Divorce, marital separation and jail term follow. This scale has been shown to be applicable to both developing and Western countries. (6: p.497)

(A19) **False.** There are seven primary mental abilities: spatial, perceptual speed, numerical reasoning, verbal meaning, word fluency, memory and inductive reasoning. (1: p.591)

(A20) **False.** Attachment is usually from infant to mother, whereas bonding is usually from mother to infant. (3: p.46)

(A21) **False.** Only psychological symptoms of depression are rated. It has 10 items rated on a four-point scale by an interviewer. (10: p.68)

(A22) **True.** Proximity allows interaction. (1: p.401)

(A23) **True.** (6: pp.495–6)

(A24) **True.** This is an example of a visual illusion. It is a room which is viewed by an observer through a peephole. He is therefore not aware that the right-hand corner is twice the distance of the left-hand corner. Thus the same objects seen in the former look surprisingly much bigger when seen in the left-hand corner. This is because the observer does not correct for the extra distance as would normally happen, because he has assumed that he is looking at a normal room. (6: pp.177–8)

(A25) **False.** It is only suitable for rating severe psychiatric illness. It is a well-standardised, observer-rated scale for measuring the severity of psychiatric symptoms, and it has subscores for affective, psychotic and negative symptoms. (10: p.68)

(A26) **False.** It is a symptom of non-dominant parietal lobe damage. (2: p.19)

(A27) **True.** (7: p.61)

(A28) **True.** (5: p.56)

(A29) **False.** This is punishment. Negative reinforcement increases a behaviour by removing an aversive stimulus. Positive reinforcement increases a behaviour by giving a positive stimulus (i.e. reward). Note that a 'punisher' can act as a negative reinforcer if it is removed from a situation. (5: pp.5–6)

(A30) **False.** There is no law of dissimilarity, but a law of similarity. Other laws include those of proximity, continuity and closure. (5: p.11)

(A31) **True.** It is also associated with attention-seeking and aggressive behaviour, language delay, dwarfed growth and bonding difficulties. (3: p.47)

(A32) **False.** It occurs when the leader is prominent and opinionated. (1: p.389)

(A33) **True.** (6: p.406)

(A34) **False.** It is arbitrary inference – that is, making conclusions in the absence of evidence. Other cognitive distortions are magnification, minimisation, personalisation, selective abstraction and over-generalisation. (2: p.307)

(A35) **True.** And also equivalent to interpreting dreams in adults. (5: p.167)

(A36) **True.** This is a mother who responds appropriately to her baby, enabling the development of the baby's true self. (5: p.168)

(A37) **False.** Mahler's theory proposed three stages: the autistic phase (with the neonate as a self-contained unit), the symbiotic phase (where the infant begins to realise that he or she is an individual, yet still remains enmeshed within the mother's self) and separation–individuation, which is subdivided into four stages, namely differentiation (4 to 8 months), practising (9 to 18 months), rapprochement (18 to 24 months) and 'on the road to object constancy'. (2: p.564)

(A38) **True.** As is inadequate ego strength (indicated by a history of repeated suicide attempts, gross DSH or violence to others, drug and alcohol addiction and serious psychosomatic conditions) and the incapacity to form and/or sustain relationships. (16: p.192)

(A39) **False.** It is associated with Arthur Janov. Reich is associated with bioenergetics, a precursor of yoga. (16: pp.181–2)

(A40) **False.** He is associated with analysis 'through the group'. Bion and Ezriel are associated with analysis 'of the group', and Wolfe and Schwarz are associated with analysis 'in the group'. The latter is similar to individual therapy, but takes place in a group setting. Analysis 'of the group' is when the therapist analyses group dynamics, and analysis 'through the group' is when the group analyses itself. (16: pp.123–5)

(A41) **True.** The remaining foci are disputes (arguments) and deficits (implying a lack of relationships). (16: pp.164–5)

(A42) **True.** (16: p.101)

(A43) **True.** Minuchin is associated with structural family therapy, and Haley is associated with strategic family therapy. (16: pp.146–7)

(A44) **True.** 5HT is an indolealkylamine. Epinephrine and nor-epinephrine are also catecholamines. (3: pp.153, 158)

(A45) **True.** In addition to drowsiness, dizziness, ataxia, headache and confusion. (9)

(A46) **True.** (9)

(A47) **False.** They have been reported with both drugs. (9)

(A48) **True.** It may cause a paradoxical increase in aggression. (9)

(A49) **True.** As it is structurally different. (9)

(A50) **False.** It does so by acting as an antagonist at $alpha_2$ receptors, resulting in increased norepinephrine release. It is also an $alpha_1$, H_1, $5HT_{2A}$ and M_1 antagonist. (10: p.690)

(A51) **False.** There is no effect on EEG at therapeutic doses. At high/toxic levels there are increased delta and theta waves. Barbiturates and benzodiazepines increase beta and delta waves but decrease alpha waves. (2: p.598)

(A52) **False.** It is an active metabolite of imipramine and lofepramine. (2: p.610) (17: p.326)

(A53) **True.** As do all phenothiazines. (9)

(A54) **False.** Other side-effects include sleep disturbance, GI disorders, headache, restlessness, agitation, paraesthesia, dry mouth, oedema and (rarely) raised liver enzymes. (9)

(A55) **True.** Barbiturates, which also have the same action, do so by increasing the length of time for which the associated chloride channel is open. (25: p.229)

(A56) **False.** They are all metabotropic. Other metabotropic receptors include the $GABA_B$, muscarinic acetylcholine, 5HT (except $5HT_3$) and dopamine receptors. Ion channels include $GABA_A$, $5HT_3$, NMDA and nicotinic acetylcholine receptors. (3: pp.164, 165, 168, 170)

(A57) **False.** Although it does cause these symptoms, it inhibits acetaldehyde dehydrogenase, resulting in the accumulation of acetaldehyde. With large doses of alcohol, arrhythmias, hypotension and collapse may even occur. It is recommended that individuals are alcohol free for at least 24 hours before treatment is initiated. (5: p.348) (9)

(A58) **True.** As is amisulpiride. (10: pp.666, 696, 705)

(A59) **True.** Maprotiline is a quadricyclic antidepressant with moderate antihistaminergic effects, but less anticholinergic effects than imipramine. (10: p.679)

(A60) **True.** As may lithium-induced weight gain. Both are side-effects at therapeutic doses. (9)

(A61) **False.** Urinary retention is a peripheral antimuscarinic side-effect, as are blurred vision, dry mouth, constipation and memory disturbance. However, postural hypotension is mediated by alpha$_1$-epinephric receptors. (11: p.220)

(A62) **False.** It is synthesised by glutamic acid decarboxylase. GABA is the main inhibitory neurotransmitter in the CNS. (11: p.312)

(A63) **False.** The reverse is true. The severity of renal impairment is usually expressed in terms of GFR (glomerular filtration rate), which is usually measured by creatinine clearance. (12: pp.39, 40, 47)

(A64) **True.** In addition to antagonistic activity at 5HT, muscarinic and alpha$_1$ receptors. (25: p.290)

(A65) **False.** Caffeine can increase it by up to 60%. (8: p.249)

(A66) **False.** It is greatest between 2 and 6 weeks. (12: pp.39, 40, 47)

(A67) **True.** 1 unit of alcohol is equivalent to approximately 8 grams of alcohol. This equates to half a pint of ordinary-strength beer, a glass of wine or a single measure of spirits. (10: p.540)

(A68) **True.** This figure is lower than in other European countries, such as France and Germany, where it is closer to 30%. (10: p.541)

(A69) **True.** It is also known as ecstasy. It is a synthetic drug and is classified in DSM-IV as a hallucinogen. It increases the release of dopamine and 5HT. (10: p.575)

(A70) **True.** As is memory impairment. (2: p.342) (13: p.289)

(A71) **False.** Although it may occur in schizophrenia. It can also occur in organic states, typically frontal lobe lesions. (13: p.158)

(A72) **True.** The patient loses the feeling of familiarity with himself, in addition to experiencing a loss of emotion. (13: p.233)

(A73) **True.** Asyndesis is a lack of adequate connection between two consecutive thoughts. It was described by Cameron. (13: p.160)

(A74) **True.** They occur in Ganser's syndrome. (13: p.173)

(A75) **False.** Individuals can speak, read and write but do not understand speech (even though their hearing is not affected). This is a form of agnosia – a lack of recognition of the spoken word. (13: p.176)

(A76) **False.** The opposite is true. Characteristic symptoms are those that occur frequently in a defined condition but also in other conditions. Discriminating symptoms occur commonly in a defined condition, but rarely in others. (10: pp.92–3)

(A77) **True.** The main symptoms are excessive and disabling fatigue in addition to exhaustion after minimal physical or mental exertion. (10: p.469)

(A78) **True.** These are hallucinations of muscle or joint sense. Other types of tactile hallucinations are superficial (affecting skin) and visceral (affecting inner organs). (13: p.106)

(A79) **True.** Panoramic recall occurs when it is felt that long periods of one's life are being rapidly re-enacted. (13: p.70)

(A80) **True.** Other important organic causes of anxiety include hyperthyroidism, hyperventilation and alcohol withdrawal. (10: p.478)

(A81) **True.** In ICD-10, emotionally unstable personality disorder is divided into borderline and impulsive types. (10: p.169)

(A82) **False.** Formication, seen in cocaine intoxication and alcohol withdrawal, is a type of superficial tactile hallucination in which there is a sensation of tiny animals or insects crawling over the body or just underneath the skin. It is often associated with delusions of infestation. (13: p.107)

(A83) **False.** They are explained by isolation, regression and reaction formation. (10: p.178)

(A84) **False.** Only naming is affected. Individuals are unable to name objects, although they may be able to describe them. Speech is fluent. (13: p.178) (15: p.17)

(A85) **False.** They occur in subjective space, although they may be vivid and have a definite outline. (13: pp.109–11)

(A86) **True.** Obsessional symptoms are resisted unsuccessfully, they are unpleasantly repetitive, and the thought of carrying out the act is not pleasurable. (13: p.329)

(A87) **False.** Content is determined by the individual's environmental, social and cultural background, whereas the form of beliefs (whether delusional, obsessional or overvalued idea) is dictated by the type of illness. (13: p.131)

(A88) **True.** (13: p.335)

(A89) **False.** They usually last for less than 30 minutes. (13: p.106)

(A90) **False.** By definition, these are abnormal beliefs that are neither delusional nor obsessional but are so preoccupying that they dominate the individual's life. Unlike obsessional thoughts, they are egosyntonic and are invariably acted upon. (13: p.143)

(A91) **False.** This is macropsia. In dysmegalopsia, objects appear larger on one side than on the other. In micropsia, objects seem smaller than their actual size. (13: p.94)

(A92) **False.** It is another term for acute schizophrenia-like psychotic disorder. This refers to the acute onset (within 2 weeks) of stable schizophrenic symptoms, but with a duration of less than 1 month. If symptoms persist for longer than this, the diagnosis should be changed to schizophrenia. (14)

(A93) **True.** Normal perception is followed by the delusional significance that is attached to this. (13: p.125)

(A94) **False.** The reverse is true. (13: p.346)

(A95) **True.** Functional hallucinations occur simultaneously with a normal perception, both being in the same modality (e.g. an auditory hallucination in association with a sound). The normal perception is required to produce the hallucination. This differs from reflex hallucinations, where a stimulus in one sensory modality produces a hallucination in another (e.g. *hearing* running water causes a *feeling* of pain in the legs). (13: pp.112–13)

(A96) **False.** The Masquerade syndrome is a hypochondriacal social phobia associated with separation anxiety in children who have required long-term medical treatment for serious illness. The illness from which they have recovered is used as an excuse not to leave home. Somatisation disorder (Briquet's syndrome) is a polysymptomatic, polysystemic, chronic hypochondriacal neurosis. (13: pp.241–68)

(A97) **False.** Although the complaint is made by the subject in relation to others, it is not usually based upon the opinion of others. Dysmorphophobia usually takes the form of an overvalued idea. (13: pp.241–68)

(A98) **False.** Clouding of consciousness does occur. Epileptic automatisms are actions that an individual is unaware of performing during or after an epileptic fit (e.g. lip smacking). Muscle tone and posture are retained, and there is amnesia for the event. They are most commonly seen in temporal lobe epilepsy. (13: p.47)

(A99) **False.** Gender describes the lifelong state or category of an organism, whereas sex describes its physical manifestation. (13: p.272)

(A100) **True.** This is a well-recognised feature of mania. (13: p.53)

(A101) **False.** It is not associated with catalepsy (a catatonic symptom) but with cataplexy (sudden loss of muscle tone provoked by strong emotions). It is also associated with hypnopompic hallucinations. (13: p.58)

(A102) **False.** It is usually associated with histrionic and antisocial personality disorder. It is also known as fluent plausible lying. (13: p.72)

(A103) **False.** This is organic hallucinosis not due to toxic substances. (14)

(A104) **True.** This can be a normal phenomenon as well as occurring in psychiatric disorders. (13: p.73)

(A105) **True.** There are often also prominent anankastic features in the individual's underlying personality. (14)

(A106) **False.** Bestiality (zoophilia) is sexual intercourse with animals. Subjects usually have limited intellectual ability and restricted social outlet, with easy access to animals. Exhibition-ists are usually passive and inadequate men. (13: p.277)

(A107) **True.** Catatonia is a state of increased muscle tone at rest, which is abolished by voluntary activity and hence differ-entiated from extrapyramidal rigidity. (13: p.364)

(A108) **False.** It occurs in response to an external stimulus and is reinforced by success. (13: p.349)

(A109) **False.** They are coordinated. (13: p.369)

(A110) **True.** Pseudodepressed type is characterised by apathy and lack of initiative. Pseudopsychopathic type is characterised by disinhibition, impulsivity and antisocial behaviour. (20: p.965)

(A111) **False.** Personality disturbance may occur in temporal lobe lesions, but is usually associated with intellectual and neuro-logical deficits. (20: p.965)

(A112) **False.** Working memory is preserved, whereas new learning (secondary memory) is severely impaired. Causes of amnesic syndrome include nutritional deficiency, infection, head injury, anoxia, vascular lesions and deep midline tumours. (20: p.966)

(A113) **False.** This describes transvestism. In transsexualism, wear-ing clothing of the opposite sex occurs without genital excitement. (13: p.274)

(A114) **False.** Astereognosis and agraphaesthesia are impairments of the *interpretation* of touch perception. Anterior parietal lobe lesions encroach on primary sensory cortex to cause contralateral cortical sensory loss in which perception of pain, temperature, touch or vibration is intact but interpret-ation is impaired. (20: p.968)

(A115) **False.** Around 50% do. Predictors of repetition of DSH include the number of previous episodes of DSH, personality disorder, history of violence, alcoholism, being unmarried and belonging to social class V. (17: p.155)

(A116) **True.** They are applied to the non-dominant hemisphere. (20: p.974)

(A117) **True.** People with good social skills may continue to function relatively better than the socially isolated or sensory deprived. (10: p.405)

(A118) **False.** It is variable, chronic and fluctuating. (14)

(A119) **True.** Subcortical dementia is characterised by slowness of thought, difficulty with complex sequential intellectual tasks and impoverishment of affect and personality. Language, calculation and learning are preserved. Cortical dysfunction includes early, prominent impairments of memory, word-finding and visuospatial abilities. (10: p.407)

(A120) **False.** A 'probable' diagnosis can be made, provided that the clinical symptoms are typical and no alternative diagnosis is plausible. (14)

(A121) **True.** Personality disorders are not mutually exclusive – there is considerable overlap in symptoms. (13: p.381)

(A122) **False.** Dissociative loss of vision or sensation is more common than both dissociative deafness and anosmia. Visual loss is rarely total; more often there is loss of acuity and blurred (or tunnel) vision. (14)

(A123) **True.** There is an impaired capacity to appreciate others' feelings, particularly how one's own actions affect others' feelings. (13: p.383)

(A124) **True.** This is calm acceptance of serious disability, which may be striking, but is not universal in dissociative disorders of movement and sensation. It may also be seen in normal individuals facing serious physical illness. (14)

(A125) **False.** They are characteristic in anankastic PD. (13: p.387)

(A126) **True.** It is performed during the day. The onset of REM less than 10 minutes after the beginning of sleep, and occurring more than twice during the period of sleep, are diagnostic. (17: p.208)

(A127) **False.** After entering sleep, there is a sequential progression through stages 1, 2, 3 and 4, followed by a return to stages 3 and 2 and then REM sleep. This cycle is repeated several times throughout the night. (15: p.149)

(A128) **True.** (2: p.301)

(A129) **False.** They contribute more to relapse than to onset. (2: p.118)

(A130) **False.** Sleep spindles and K complexes occur in stage 2. In stage 1, alpha activity diminishes to less than 50%, giving way to low-voltage delta activity. (2: p.536) (15: p.148)

(A131) **False.** Relapse rates are similar. (8: p.122)

(A132) **False.** More than 50% do. The condition is more frequent in primigravidae and in those who suffer from premenstrual tension. (10: p.501)

(A133) **False.** Although this is true of DSM-IV, in ICD-10 it is classified in the section on schizophrenia. (2: p.298)

EMI 1

(A134) **G.** (7: p.61)

(A135) **F.** (7: p.59)

(A136) **D.** (7: p.59)

(A137) **E.** (7: p.60)

(A138) **C.** (7: p.61)

(A139) **A.** (7: p.61)

EMI 2

(A140) **A.** This rarely persists in later life as a social anxiety disorder. (7: p.70)

(A141) **E.** (7: p.73)

The following are Erikson's stages of psychosocial development:

Infancy	Trust versus mistrust
2–3 years	Autonomy versus shame and doubt
3–5 years	Initiative versus guilt
6–11 years	Industry versus inferiority
Adolescence	Identity versus role confusion
Early adulthood	Intimacy versus isolation
Middle age	Generativity versus stagnation
Old age	Integrity versus despair.

(A142) **C.** Confidence is considered to be a successful outcome at this stage. (3: p.43) (7: p.73)

(A143) **D.** Gender labelling is achieved by 3 years. (7: p.72)

(A144) **F.** As is fear of examinations. (5: p.73)

EMI 3

(A145) **A.** He emphasised social factors in development, such as sibling rivalry (as an attempt to deal with feelings of inferiority), organ inferiority and masculine protest (in women, as a reaction to their inferior position in society). (2: p.562)

(A146) **C.** He emphasised the collective unconscious and the archetypes within it (e.g. the Hero and the Great Mother). These archetypes are manifested as symbols in dreams or disturbed states of mind. (5: p.165)

(A147) **H.** The manifest content of a dream is what is remembered after waking up, whereas the latent content is the meaning of the dream. The latent content is hidden and can be bypassed by free association during therapy. (16: p.13)

(A148) **D.** He developed client-centred therapy. According to Rogers, every individual aims for consistency between their self-concept and their experiences. (2: p.90)

(A149) **I.** Pairing is when individuals in a group form procreative groups, leading to the 'birth of a person or idea that would provide salvation'. Other basic assumptions are dependence and fight/flight; these hinder the group's progress. (2: p.562)

(A150) **F.** A child must pass through three phases – autistic, symbiotic and separation–individuation – to achieve object constancy. (2: p.564)

EMI 4

(A151) **C.** This, together with mitgehen, automatic obedience and advertence, is a symptom of excessive cooperation. (13: p.365)

(A152) **B.** (13: p.365)

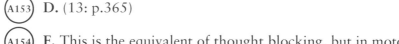

(A153) **D.** (13: p.365)

(A154) **F.** This is the equivalent of thought blocking, but in motor actions. (13: p.365)

(A155) **I.** (13: p.364)

(A156) **A.** In contrast, aversion is when the patient turns away from the examiner. It is an example of opposition (a negative response to the examiner, which may also manifest as muteness). (13: p.365)

EMI 5

Reference for all (14)

(A157) **G.**

(A158) **H.**

(A159) **E.**

(A160) **A.**

(A161) **B.**

(A162) **H.**

EMI 6

(A163) **E, F, G, H.** Others include short duration of illness and being married. (10: p.364)

(A164) **A, B, C, D, I.** Others include social isolation and poor compliance with medication. (10: p.364)

(A165) **I.** And a short history. (10: p.448)

I. The best predictor of future course is the history of previous episodes. (10: p.305)

EMI 7

 E, F. This is the commonest psychiatric disorder following head injury. Other symptoms include fatigue, dizziness, sexual dysfunction, mild cognitive impairment, sleep disturbance, irritability, anxiety and depression. (2: p.401)

 C, G. The psychiatric sequelae of CVAs include depression, cognitive impairment, personality change, anxiety, emotional lability and catastrophic reaction (the latter particularly in left frontal lobe strokes). Symptoms include upper motor neuron motor signs, hemiplegia, loss or disturbance of speech and focal neurological signs. The commonest cause is thromboembolism of the middle cerebral artery. (10: p.330) (21: p.354)

 B, H. Recurrent head injury in boxers leads to subcortical dementia with Parkinsonian symptoms, cerebellar symptoms, irritability, explosive behaviour, morbid jealousy, pathological intoxication, paranoia and personality change. (2: p.402)

 A, J. It causes frontal lobe symptoms including personality change, perseveration, aphasia, anosmia, palilalia, ipsilateral optic atrophy and aspontaneity. (5: p.21)

 D, I. Other symptoms include fatigue, generalised musculoskeletal aches and pains, abdominal discomfort, diarrhoea and a bad taste. In more severe cases there can be a motor peripheral neuropathy resulting in wrist and foot drop, anaemia, renal tubular damage, blue lines on the gum margins and radiopathic lead lines on long bones. (23: p.170)

EMI 8

(A172)   **G.** This woman is not disturbed and drugs (e.g. lorazepam) can potentially cause ataxia and falls. (9)

(A173)   **A.** TCAs would be contraindicated, as their anticholinergic effect can exacerbate benign prostate hypertrophy. (9)

(A174)   **E.** Although there is a possibility she may have Lewy body dementia, a small dose of antipsychotic medication can be used with great caution. (4: p.505) (5: p.561)

(A175)   **B.** Urgent ECT is indicated. (5: p.557)

EMI 9

(A176)   **F.** Cocaine has a stimulant and euphoric effect. It produces tachycardia, increased temperature and blood pressure, dilated pupils and convulsions. Toxic effects include muscle twitching, nausea, vomiting, hyperpyrexia and cardiac arrhythmias. The psychiatric implications of cocaine use can be divided into four stages, namely euphoria, dysphoria upon craving, hallucinosis and psychosis. (4: p.618)

(A177)   **D.** Cannabis can cause acute anxiety. Paranoid, schizophreniform reactions and hypomanic features may occur in the predisposed. The 'flashbacks', similar to those experienced after LSD use, are relatively frequent and more common in individuals who have previously used LSD. Craving and psychological dependency are rare. On abrupt withdrawal in heavy users, irritability, weakness, insomnia and anorexia may occur. (4: p.613)

(A178)   **H.** LSD use is not associated with physical dependence or withdrawal symptoms. It causes dilated pupils, piloerection, increased temperature and tendon reflexes, muscle twitching and tremors, somnolence, giddiness and mood disturbance (euphoria, anxiety, withdrawal or passivity). Perceptual distortions are common and mainly consist of visual hallucinations and synaesthesia. (4: p.620)

(A179) **K.** The withdrawal syndrome reaches a peak on the third or fourth day after abstinence from opiates. Although unpleasant, it is not life-threatening. Other symptoms include craving, anxiety, sweating, goose pimples, muscle twitching, vomiting, diarrhoea, tachycardia and hypertension. (4: p.612)

EMI 10

(A180) **F, H, K.** (4: p.453)

(A181) **A, D, I.** A score of greater than 7 on the Hachinski scale suggests vascular dementia. The following are assessed: abrupt onset, step-wise deterioration, fluctuating course, nocturnal confusion, relative preservation of personality, depression, somatic complaints, emotional incontinence, history of hypertension, history of stroke, evidence of associated arteriosclerosis, focal neurological signs and focal neurological symptoms. (4: p.453)

(A182) **B, G, J.** (4: p.460)

References

1 Gross R (2001) *Psychology: the science of mind and behaviour.* Hodder & Stoughton, London.

2 Wright P, Stern J and Phelan M (2001) *Core Psychiatry.* Saunders, Edinburgh.

3 Malhi G (2002) *Examination Notes in Psychiatry: Basic Sciences.* Arnold, London.

4 Lishman WA (1998) *Organic Psychiatry: the psychological consequences of cerebral disorder.* Blackwell Science, Oxford.

5 Puri B and Hall A (2004) *Revision Notes in Psychiatry.* Hodder Arnold, London.

6 Smith E, Nolen-Hoeksema S, Fredrickson B *et al.* (2003) *Atkinson and Hilgard's Introduction to Psychology.* Wadsworth, Belmont, CA.

7 Leung W and Passmore K (2001) *Essential Notes for the MRCPsych Part 1.* Petroc Press, Newbury.

8 Taylor D, Paton C and Kerwin R (2003) *The Maudsley 2003 Prescribing Guidelines.* Martin Dunitz, London.

9 British Medical Association and the Royal Pharmaceutical Society of Great Britain (2004) *British National Formulary. Number 47.* British Medical Association and the Royal Pharmaceutical Society of Great Britain, London.

10 Gelder M, Mayou R and Cowen P (2001) *Shorter Oxford Textbook of Psychiatry.* Oxford University Press, Oxford.

11 Stahl S and Muntner N (2000) *Essential Psychopharmacology: neuroscientific basis and practical applications.* Cambridge University Press, Cambridge.

12 Cookson J, Taylor D and Katona C (2002) *Use of Drugs in Psychiatry.* Gaskell, London.

13 Sims A (2003) *Symptoms in the Mind.* Saunders, London.

14 World Health Organization (1992) *The ICD-10 Classification of Mental and Behavioural Disorders: clinical descriptions and diagnostic guidelines.* World Health Organization, Geneva.

15 Malhi G, Matharu M and Hale A (2000) *Neurology for Psychiatrists.* Martin Dunitz, London.

16 Bateman A, Brown D and Pedder J (2002) *Introduction to Psychotherapy.* Brunner-Routledge, Hove.

17 Buckley P, Bird J and Harrison G (2001) *Examination Notes in Psychiatry.* Arnold, London.

18 American Psychiatric Association (1994) *Diagnostic and Statistical Manual of Mental Disorders, Fourth Edition (DSM-IV).* American Psychiatric Association, Washington, DC.

19 Johnstone E, Freeman C and Zealley A (eds) (1998) *Companion to Psychiatric Studies.* Churchill Livingstone, Edinburgh.

20 Stein G and Wilkinson G (1998) *Seminars in General Adult Psychiatry. Volume 2.* Gaskell, London.

21 Longmore M, Wilkinson IB and Rajagopalan S (2004) *Oxford Handbook of Clinical Medicine.* Oxford University Press, New York.

22 Kumar P and Clark M (2004) *Clinical Medicine.* Saunders, Philadelphia, PA.

23 Haslett C, Chilviers ER, Boon NA *et al.* (eds) (2002) *Davidson's Principles and Practice of Medicine.* Churchill Livingstone, Philadelphia, PA.

24 National Institute for Clinical Excellence (2003) *Guidance on the Use of Electroconvulsive Therapy. Technology Appraisal Guidance 59.* National Institute for Clinical Excellence, London.

25 Leonard B (2003) *Fundamentals of Psychopharmacology.* John Wiley & Sons, Chichester.

Index

(q) refer to question locators; (a) refer to answer locators